real
Gorgeous

real Gorgeous

The truth about body and beauty

KAZ COOKE

W. W. NORTON & COMPANY

NEW YORK   LONDON

Cover: *Our radiant covergirl, Hermione the Modern Girl, is wearing a frock from the Burnie op-shop. Hair by accident. Styling: hardly likely. Makeup: old lipstick from the bottom of her handbag from which the label has worn off. There may have been eyebrow pencil involvement, although this is by no means certain. Shoes: model's own. Underpants: yes. Signature fragrance: Eau de Faff, by Serge-Penelope Froufrou de Prohibitively expensif. Photographed exclusively for* Real Gorgeous *by the Mervyn Purvis Agency, Paris, Rome, New York, Dili and Marble Bar. All rights reserved.*

The text of this book is composed in Bembo, with display type set in Ad Lib, Camelia, and Clearface. This book was composed on desktop using Adobe Pagemaker 5.0 by Justine Burkat Trubey. Manufacturing by the Courier Companies, Inc.

Library of Congress Cataloging-in-Publication Data

Cooke, Kaz, 1962–
    Real gorgeous : the truth about body and beauty / by Kaz Cooke.
        p.   cm.
    Originally published: St. Leonards NSW, Australia : Allen & Unwin, 1994.
    Includes bibliographical references and index.
    ISBN 0-393-31355-7 (pbk.)
    1. Body image. 2. Beauty, Personal—Psychological aspects.
3. Self-esteem. 4. Feminine beauty (Aesthetics) I. Title.
BF697.5.B63C66 1996
613'.04244—dc20   95-13464
                                                                              CIP

W. W. Norton & Company, Inc., 500 Fifth Avenue, New York, NY 10110
W. W. Norton & Company Ltd., 10 Coptic Street, London WC1A 1PU

1 2 3 4 5 6 7 8 9 0

Contents

Acknowledgements

Chris ("of all the places I've been, libraries are the sexiest") Pip was the researcher on *Real Gorgeous*: my thanks to her for panting amongst the shelves, the interviews with research subjects, and her efficient collating and presentation of the right stuff.

For help in supplying, interpreting, and checking information, thanks are due to Penelope Goward, the Australasian College of Dermatologists and its swag of helpful experts, Dr. Neil Hewson, Sue Noy, the Alcohol and Drug Foundation, the Anorexia and Bulimia Association of Victoria, the Royal Prince Alfred Hospital Eating Disorders Clinic, Rosemary Stanton, Ruth Trickey, and Penelope Tree.

Thank you also to the staff of the *Age* newspaper library in Melbourne and the Condé Nast library in New York, to the students who copied the graffiti on college and university toilet walls about body image in response to my letter published in campus newspapers, and to the editors of the magazines which printed my request for letters about body image.

I am particularly grateful to all women who wrote to me with their thoughts on many issues. Each was useful. Excerpts from these letters appear as edited quotes throughout the book. All names have been changed.

Cynthia Heimel quotes from *Get Your Tongue Out of My Mouth, I'm Kissing You Goodbye* (New York: Ballantine, 1993).

Victoria Wood quotes from *Mens Sana in Thingummy Doodah* (London: Mandarin, 1993) and *Up to You Porky* (London: Mandarin, 1993).

Extract from "Magazine" episode reproduced from *Absolutely Fabulous* by Jennifer Saunders with the permission of BBC Enterprises Limited.

The book you hold was culled from a wee mountain of information, with a great deal of help and support. Thank you Chris Pip,

Julie Gibbs, Anna Dollard, Jenna Mead, Mary Sinclair, Sharon Connolly, Mark Davis, Foong Ling Kong, Glenda Jones, Philippa Hawker, and Lisby Gore.

And to Susan Wyndham, for "Americanizing" where it was needed. Metric measurements in quotes have been silently changed to American measures (e.g., 5'9" instead of 175 cm, 138 pounds instead of 63 kilograms).

Introduction

We need something that will cheer up anybody who has "the uglies." Something to reassure all certifiably gorgeous girls and women that they are not Space Porkers from Hell.

We need the facts which will make us RELAX, not the overwrought opinions that send us fleeing to stupid diets, insane overexercising, and mirror-misery. We want to find out how to stop seeing our bodies as the enemy. And hey, let's face it, we wouldn't mind a laugh while we're at it.

We need some help with self-esteem which cuts through the mixed messages of magazine articles called "Love Your Own Body" illustrated only by professionally lit retouched photos of a size-8, six-foot-tall, 13-year-old aerobics instructor-model wearing a frilly baby-doll dress, platform thigh-high boots, and a terminally bored expression.

We need to get away from too many dry statistics, relentless academic essays, incomprehensible diagrams, and scientific formulas that don't seem to relate to real life. We need stuff which frees us to make up our own minds. And maybe cartoons would be a lot more fun than endless pictures of models.

We need a book that isn't just about theory but about action: *how* to break out of the useless dieting cycle, *how* to deal with dorks who make comments about our appearance, *how* to accept a natural womanly shape, whether tall, small, thin, or rounded.

We'd like to know how to avoid and deal with eating disorders, and what we can eat without panicking. We want the truth about skin care products: which cheap ones work and which ones advertise using pretend science, fancy French, and straight-out lies. We want to have fun with clothes and makeup, not feel that we have to spend a fortune of stuff to blindly follow fashion.

We need to know why cosmetic surgery is not about simple "nips and tucks," but pain, and gouging, and self-hatred, and desperation that has other answers than the knife. We'd like to be able to laugh off the *Allure* magazine suggestion that face-lift bandages might become a "fashion trend."

We need some information that, unlike magazines, isn't influenced by advertising. A book that isn't trying to sell you anything except more self-confidence and the truth. Something that we can always open to remind ourselves that it's okay that we have different shapes, different sizes, and different skin. (Not to mention the odd tuft of body hair.) A book that we can run to any time we feel like screaming at the very sight of a cakie thing.

In short, we need a book that gathers all this stuff together, combines the facts and the fun, and gives us some options about where to look for more help if we need it.

I couldn't find such a book, so I had to write one. Here it is.

It stayed at the top of best-seller lists in Australia for months, and filled my in-tray with mail from grateful Australian girls and women, saying they felt good about their bodies at last, able to repel the body police with a single glance, and leap tall chocolate binges with a single bound...well, you know what I mean.

I hope that Americans will gain the same sense of fun and freedom in reading *Real Gorgeous*. We've "translated" it to produce an American edition more relevant to you, but kept the gist and the jokes (hurrah, or should I say woooo, woooooo?). As we say in Australia—go for it (or perhaps we got that from you). Enjoy.

Kaz Cooke
Real Gorgeous

real Gorgeous

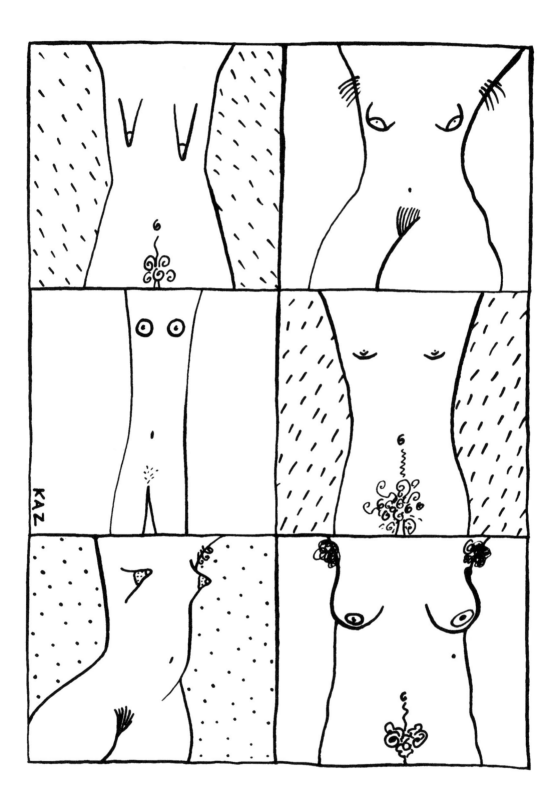

chapter one

Shapes and Sizes

In the beginning

Whoopsie, where did these curvy bits come from? Like a little old caterpillar programmed to become a butterfly, our grown-up shapes are already decided before we are born. When we get to puberty, we find out what kind of a butterfly we are.

The teenage years: who needs 'em? Is the world deliberately trying to confuse us or what? We're sitting around minding our own business and suddenly our bodies go berserk.

Our shape changes dramatically, we grow to our full height, start periods, gain extra breast tissue and other fat deposits in our lower body. (It lasts from about age 10 until about 15, although the changes sometimes don't finish until your early 20s.)

There's the arrival of hair in previously bald places. Very often one breast grows larger than the other for some time until the other one catches up, but the right one often ends up slightly larger. Vaginal lips enlarge. There's extra sweating.

Everyone gets terribly embarrassed and wants to hide their bits. Nobody feels much like a beautiful butterfly. Sometimes it feels more like being a squished caterpillar.

In many other cultures these rites of passage are celebrated with ceremony, which would seem a more healthy way of going about it. This is the sort of time any reasonable society would send its children on a long holiday, complete with instructions on how to be an adult and why you're still gorgeous. Instead they give you exams. Weird.

The changes happen differently for each person, at different speeds. Sometimes, people go BOING. On average, girls start their changes two or three years before boys. Hormonal changes often induce pimples as well (thank you so much, I think I'd rather just have the hips). Girls will add 25 to 40 pounds to their body weight during this time and grow to maximum height with a few more pounds to come before they turn 20 or so.

Before puberty, girls have 10 to 15 percent more fat than boys. After puberty, they have 20 to 30 percent more fat than boys. Both sexes have a growth spurt, the male one being mostly in muscle and lean tissue, the female in fat tissue.

Anyway, the point is, we put on more flesh on our hips while boys lose it. Suddenly "oh my GOD" you think you're getting fat. You're getting bigger in all the areas you've heard women complain about and loathe and pinch with rueful expressions. But you're not getting fat at all. You're becoming a woman. The much-criticised pear shape is natural. When girls become women, fat is deposited around their hips and stomach in preparation for fertility and protection for the uterus, should you decide to avail yourself of its possibilities.

> Being thin ain't all it's cracked up to be. I'm 18, five feet four, and 99 to 106 pounds and size five. I'm a very light frame and I'm one of those people who can eat bucketloads of food and not put on an ounce. It's almost impossible to get clothes that fit properly. Get sick, and forget it, I soon resemble a skeleton, my hipbones protrude, as well as every other bone it seems. It's really scary to drop 10 or 12 pounds when you're already thin. It does get embarrassing to hear all those girls with what I consider perfectly healthy, gorgeous bodies envying my figure. I never see their size, I see past their body shape to look at what's inside them. It's our minds that make our bodies either embarrassing or acceptable. I've had so many guys comment on the fact that it's nice to see a girl enjoy her food.
>
> Kimberley, 18

Breasts are also made up mostly of fat tissue. The extent of these changes is governed by genetics. (You may be told you have your auntie's breasts, and wonder if you should give them back.) Your eventual shape, programmed into you before you were born, will be a different cocktail of genes from your sisters and, of course, your brothers.

Me

3 parts Dad - - - -

Dash of Mum - - -

2 shakes - - -
Grandma

10 ml - - - -
Aunty
Judy

GeNe cockᵼAiL SHaKeR

Girls who mature early may be shorter, heavier for their height, and have shorter legs than girls who mature later. These girls are hit with a double whammy of feeling changed and different before their thinner, taller friends, and also less like the thin ideal they may feel they have to conform to. Others may be "late bloomers."

Even girls with small breasts and slight hips go through the changes. They are no less women for having fewer curves. Their bodies, too, have made the necessary changes during puberty.

Some adolescent girls delay these changes by exercising too much and underfeeding themselves. Their body shapes are retarded at an earlier growth stage and the onset of periods is delayed. This is common in ballet and gymnastics students and athletes, and shamefully encouraged by some teachers. One study showed ballet dancers delayed the onset of menstruation for an average of three years.

One hundred years ago the average age to begin menstruation in the well-fed parts of the world was 16. It's now between 12 ½ and 13. This is thought to be due to improved nutrition, or possibly Mars Bars.

You can't change your shape

By the time you've been through puberty, you'll know whether you're going to be tall and thin or tall and big or short and curvy. What about all those people who say you can change your shape through diet and exercise? Not true: you can change your weight overall but not the general pattern of weight distribution. What's more, your distribution of fat and muscle fibre was also programmed into you before you were born.

Fat patterns differ between people, but they are not changed by dieting. Most women who diet regain their previous body weight within two years (more on this in the diet section), and the body will return to its natural shape after excessive exercising and dieting are stopped.

In a study called "Is Body Fat Distribution Changed by Dieting?" John Garrow concluded: "With weight loss the waist-hip ratio does not change but the waist-thigh ratio decreases. This is to be expected since in obesity there is a relatively greater deposit of fat on the waist than on the thighs" (e.g., a big "beer belly").

What the man is trying to say in doctorspeak is that there is no proof that more fat is lost from one body part and not others during weight loss. In other words, you're still going to be the same shape after dieting—just lighter. And you'll still be the same shape after exercising—only leaner.

> My body is pear-shaped and I can't stand it, my hips and thighs are way too big for what I want. I've tried many different diets but can never seem to stick to them. I always end up pigging out on junk food then I feel guilty and don't eat for two or three days, hoping to lose the weight I put on. I read this can be bad for you but that doesn't bother me, I just want to lose weight.
>
> Anonymous

Another study showed that physical training may not reduce body weight (as muscle replaces fat) but could reduce the waist-hip ratio by between 3 and 6 percent: nowhere near enough to be noticeable to the naked eye. The study found that fat cells on the bottom, hips, and thighs were more difficult to reduce than the abdominal fat cells.

The fat controllers Dr. Sandra Cabot has been gaining publicity in Australia with public appearances, seminars, and her books on hormones and dieting; she is the author of *The Body Shaping Diet*. Dr. Cabot is one of many people claiming that there are four body types. Android (strong, thickset, relatively uncurvy, more "masculine," extra fat deposited above the pelvis); gynaeoid (the majority: pear-shaped, extra fat deposited on the thighs, buttocks, breasts, and later the lower abdomen); lymphatic (generalised thickening and puffiness due to fluid retention, especially in the limbs, and fat distribution all over the body: "Lymphatic women have often been 'chubby' since childhood," says Dr. Cabot); and thyroid (narrow, long-limbed, smaller-breasted with weight gain occurring first around the abdomen and upper thighs).

The problem with this sort of theory is that there are not only four different body types. There are millions, all bodies with different metabolisms, genes, environments, colouring, ways of life, culturally determined and geographically determined eating habits, all with different hormonal influences, ages, places in the cycle of life, and times in the menstrual cycle.

Now that I'm a mum I'm especially interested in mothers' figures. I look at all Demi Moore's semi-nude shots to see if she had stretch marks and a flabby stomach. And with her *Vanity Fair* cover, why didn't I look like that when I was pregnant with my second child?

Annie, 24

Because you didn't have full-body makeup, professional lighting, a day-long team of makeup and hair artists, and airbrushing and retouching of the photographs before publication. Because you don't have a team of housekeepers and nannies so you can do three to seven boring hours of gym work a day, as Demi Moore said she did following the birth of each child. Like other actresses, she has body doubles available to her for close-ups if she chooses.

Like many people living in confusing times, Dr. Cabot speaks of control. "Women want knowledge about how they can help themselves so they can get a feeling of control in their lives." It is dangerous to equate control over your life with impossible control over your body shape. Who has control over everything anyway? (And can they be stopped?!)

The Body Shaping Diet, like other books claiming to change the shape of one part of the body (*The Hip and Thigh Diet*, *The Buns Diet*), sells by claiming to be a "breakthrough in weight control." Dr. Cabot claims that the diet will get rid of cellulite. "Cellulite is unsightly," she told *Who Weekly* (it's the Australian version of *People*), which ran a cover story on her theories. "But if it doesn't concern you, don't worry about it." How encouraging.

She concludes, "[My] book is about giving women the chance of getting off their bums and eating the right food." One gets the impression that Dr. Cabot is dead against women sitting on their bums: "I am a woman who controls her life completely." Dr. Cabot admitted to being nine pounds underweight, "so busy I don't eat properly." Her co-author, an herbalist, said, "Whenever we travel together I make sure we have breakfast and dinner."

Dr. Cabot has not convinced others in the medical profession that special foods in combinations will target fat on one area of the body. She concedes that body type is genetically coded but insists, "You can lose weight in specific areas just by having the right food combinations to balance your metabolism." Her diet, for example, bans dairy foods for lymphatic (large) women and stimulants for thyroid (thin) women.

Her description of thyroid women as "the envy of all others," inclined to be "highly strung" and "prone to eating disorders like anorexia," prompted many of *Who Weekly*'s readers to write and complain that they were tall and thin, not highly strung, and certainly not prone to eating disorders. Dr. Cabot had suggested that the Princess of Wales's body shape rather than her state of mind was characteristic of bulimics.

Despite the hopes of women who read this kind of stuff, full control over your life is an impossible enough goal without expecting that you can control your hip shape as well.

Recently Australian *Cosmopolitan* ran a full-page photograph of model Naomi Campbell with the screaming headline "Is this the Perfect Body?" and answered: "Yes it probably is—the perfect combination of strength and femininity. This body belongs to supermodel Naomi Campbell but you, too, can achieve Naomi's fit, shapely look."

The magazine went on to describe "the body"—not the woman but the packaging—as "5'9" of absolute perfection. Twenty-one-year-old Naomi's body is a work of art. Her well-defined, wide shoulders and 34-inch bust taper down to a 23-inch waist and slim 34-inch hips, with a pert bottom and long, shapely legs." This erotic description was next to a picture of an oiled Naomi Campbell almost in the nude (in high heels and holding a length of shiny, red fabric) with her back to the camera and looking back over her shoulder.

"For Naomi, a superb body was a gift of nature—for the rest of us it is something that can be attained with a good diet, exercise, willpower and determination." The magazine noted that Ms. Campbell weighed only 106 pounds, with body fat of about 16 percent, almost certainly too low for regular periods, if any at all. It reported that 16 percent was "just over half that of an average woman's count of 30 percent on a typical 138-pound, 5'3" frame."

Cosmo's editor began a subsequent magazine with an apology. "Whoops did we ever get it wrong! But we're not guilty of irresponsibility as some of our readers suggested. What we are guilty of is inaccuracy. Our story put the beautiful black English model's weight at 106 pounds. When your letters began to arrive we contacted Naomi's agent in London (our article originated from there) and found that she in fact weighs in at around 120 pounds."

"As the editor of a magazine that has the glamour image *Cosmo* has," continued editor Pat Ingram, "I'm often accused of promoting an unrealistic beauty ideal. I don't believe this is true. Certainly our fashion and beauty pages feature good-looking, slim models, but they are just that, models—girls who make their living from their looks, girls who conform to society's current standards of physical female beauty. Ideally, every woman would be slim: it not only looks better, it's healthier. It's when the pursuit of *slim* becomes the obsession to be *thin* that the danger sets in" (her emphases).

Slim does NOT look better on everybody, and is not necessarily more healthy. The real danger is that naturally non-slim women are endangering their health because they're told they could have a body like Naomi Campbell through diet and exercise (and very soon I expect to be much taller, with an insolent bottom, and rather black).

British *Slimmer* magazine ran an article called "You Can Change Your Shape." They defined only three body shapes—short and round (endomorph), lean and muscly (mesomorph), or tall and bony (ectomorph). The writers of the article ("famous for books and videos") say a short, round person can become leaner, and tall, bony people who do "toning" exercises will "become more shapely." One person participating in the article who didn't like her hips had to do daily exercises, power walking three times a week, and swimming three times a week. Of course she lost weight. But there was no proof given for her, or any others, that the basic body shape had changed.

One of the strongest pushes from the shape-changing propagandists is the phrase "body sculpting," heavy exercise of the kind that changed Madonna from a fleshy dancer into a hard-bodied one. If you concentrate on one or a few muscles, and work only on them, you will get a bigger, more defined muscle. That's why skaters develop bigger thighs and weightlifters bigger arms. Going the other way—making an area smaller by losing weight only from one specific area—is virtually undocumented.

"Body shape is not simply a gift from nature," claims the headline on a Clarins cosmetics ad. "Slim, firm contours and smooth skin result from a healthy lifestyle and daily care with specific, high-performance products." These would presumably include the Contouring Body Cream and the Body Shaping Gel. The Contouring Cream does not contour, but tightens the skin while it is on, as egg white or glue does. The Body Shaping Gel does not shape your body, it is supposed to "minimise the appearance of sponginess" by plumping out the skin. The Multi Mass Massage Mitt, also advertised, is claimed to "enhance firmness and tone" but it simply irritates the skin into temporary slight swelling which then looks smoother.

Many people assume I am anorexic because I am thin. In fact I probably eat more than other girls my age because everyone is always trying to fatten me up. I eat properly and am very active, and I find it insulting to be labelled anorexic. I have never even considered dieting. And in an effort to bolster up large girls' self-esteem, we thin girls are described as scrawny, waif-like, childlike, and figureless. I may be petite, but I am every inch Woman!

Peta, 20

Remember: doctors disagree on exactly how many body types there are. But look around: there are as many as there are women. Or at least 837.

The one thing almost all of the people who say you can change your shape have in common is that they are trying to sell you something.

International Clothes Sizes

Australian	8	10	12	14	16	18	20
French	36	38	40	42	44	46	48
Italian	38	40	42	44	46	48	50
German	34	36	38	40	42	44	46
English	8	10	12	14	16	18	20
American	6	8	10	12	14	16	18
Japanese	7	9	11	13			

Clothes sizes Most clothes sizes have a variation of two inches. That means a size 12 in one label might fit you but a size 12 by another designer will feel too tight. At this point the sales assistant will say, "It's European, dear," or "It will shrink a bit when you wash it," or "No, madam, this fabric never shrinks," or "You'll grow into it," or "You can lose a couple of pounds," or "Get out of the shop, you monster." This is why elastic-waisted things are easy and why you should always try on something even if it says "free size" or "one size" or "one size fits all." (And by the way, can someone tell me why labels have "small," "medium," and "large" for women and "1," "2," and "3" for men?)

Some women's clothing companies still base their patterns on body-measurement standards set by the U.S. government in 1942 when American women were smaller and the population was less ethnically diversified than it is now. During the 1950s and 1960s, women managed to squeeze themselves into the old sizes with incredibly

Average fittings according to United States standards (in inches)

Size	6	8	10	12	14	16
						and so on up to size 22
Bust	31.5	32.5	33.5	35	36.5	38
Waist	22.5	23.5	24.5	26	27.5	29
Hip	33.5	34.5	35.5	37	38.5	40

uncomfortable whalebone corsets and scary rubber pantie girdles.

These days, the sizing system makes even less sense, so lots of clothing manufacturers have developed their own set of measurements. They also try to save time and money by making fewer sizes. So most women have trouble buying clothes and have a closet full of different sizes.

"I used to think that I was a 12, but not necessarily," says Frances Dysart, a 35-year-old New York secretary. "In more expensive designer clothes like Ellen Tracy, I can sometimes wear a 10 or even an 8."

The reason is that designers want to seduce women into buying their expensive clothes, so they "flatter" us by making us feel smaller than we really are. "Oh my GOD, I'm a size EIGHT here? Let me get my wallet! Hurrah! My credit card is yours!" Few designers make

allowances for the fact that many women have different sizes within their own body—for example, a size-16 skirt and a size-12 blouse.

"In the U.S. there is not a standard size 8," says Professor Ingrid Johnson, chair of the textile development and marketing department at Parsons School of Design in New York. "A Calvin Klein 8 is larger than if you bought a Liz Claiborne size 8 and certainly larger than if you bought a K-Mart or Walmart 8. You'd probably take a size 12 at K-Mart."

When Nancy Reagan was First Lady in the 1980s, it was well known that she wore a teeny-weeny, itsy-bitsy, haven't-had-lunch-for-three-months size 2. Millions of American women wanted to emulate her but they couldn't shrink, of course, so many manufacturers started cutting their sizes larger. "You saw more 2s and 4s in the stores, when in reality Americans are getting larger," says Professor Johnson.

There is hope! American Standards and Testing Materials, a not-for-profit group that sets standards for many industries, has formed a committee that is taking measurements of 7,000 American women of different ages and ethnic groups. Based on these Real Women, the committee hopes to establish some new, *real* fitting standards. In the meantime—don't take any notice of the size on the tag—try everything on to make sure it's positively you-sized.

In her book *Being Fat Is Not a Sin*, English writer Shelley Povey demonstrates how clothes sizes can be manipulated to make women feel flattered or estranged. The English size 14 used to be a medium, now it's a large. She says that in 1985 the Big Is Beautiful movement reported that 50 percent of British women were a size 16 and over (large). Now that message has subtly changed to 60 percent being size 14 and over. More than half of the female population were suddenly made "large" by the stroke of a pen.

Puberty was not kind. I grew taller, bigger, and spottier than everybody in sixth grade. I tried practically every weight-loss method invented. Sometimes I would lie in bed at night stupidly wishing some alien life form would kidnap me, free me of my fat (preferred alien method was by rolling down the fat off my body, like you would roll down stockings), and then return the slimmer, beautiful new me back to earth. Of course this never happened.

Susan, 24

Customer: So you haven't got anything in a size 12?

Assistant: They might have sent something by mistake. There's these....

Customer: They look a bit small to me.

Assistant: It's up to you, Porky.

Comedian Victoria Wood

Bovey points out that in 1960 Marilyn Monroe "epitomised all that was enviable to women and desirable to men. The little black dress she wore in *Some Like It Hot* was recently displayed in an exhibition of costumes. It was an outsize dress, a size 14."

The clothes you see on models, even really tall ones, are usually size 8 or 6. One model agent says of designers, "They only produce size-8 samples and a slim silhouette makes a wonderful clotheshorse." Well tie her up, give her a handful of oats, and see whether she whinnies.

Where to see normal You will see only one type of normal in the magazines and on television and in films. That's the estimated 5 percent of us, the model-shaped thin girls, with very long legs and wide shoulders. In years gone by we had actors ranging from Sophia Loren's shape to Mae West and back to feisty Katharine Hepburn and Rosalind Russell (check out the classics section at your video shop). English and Australian actors tend to have more diverse shapes but we see mostly the American ideal on our screens, which is the thinnest with the most makeup and the most fussed-over hair. It is also the most fiddled-with image, the most removed from reality, from the fake world (the planet of *Melrose Place*).

We have to start looking at the real world again as well as watching the TV and reading the magazines. If we have our head stuck in that stuff all the time our idea of what is normal gets completely out of whack because we are seeing only the Five Percent. Go see women in the shopping mall. Oh my God! Where did all these real people come from? See how differently shaped they are? See how the mothers and the women who have been through menopause look different? And if you really want to see life as it is, go and swim at a local pool or the beach or do an exercise class at a community gym, and have a look around you in the changing room. Here we are. The 95 percent. The 100 percent. All different. Real gorgeous.

Why are we told to be skinny?

The freedom theory Thinness became a symbol of reproductive freedom, independence, and youthful fun in the 1920s. The thinness ideal was born of women competing with men for jobs and opportunities: a denial of being seen as fit only for reproduction and decoration.

The health theory "Thinner" always means "healthier" and "larger" automatically means "less healthy." Tell that to the tooth fairy.

The backlash theory As women gain more political and economic power, the pressures on them to diet and be judged only by what they look like are intensified. This is part of the backlash against feminism. This theory is supported by Susan Faludi in her book *Backlash* and by Naomi Wolf in her book *The Beauty Myth*.

The fear of fat theory There is prejudice against fat people. "Excess body fat is probably the most stigmatised physical feature except skin colour, but unlike skin colour is thought to be under control," said one team of authors looking into obesity and women. From childhood people attribute other characteristics to those who are fat, including being dirty, untidy, ugly, lazy, and stupid.

The media theory The media cover the different variations of the communications industry, including press, film, and television. These media have set up an impossible, glamorous ideal and censor most other images of real women by excluding them. For example, a male reporter can be bald and fat as long as his work is satisfactory, but a woman newsreader on a commercial channel cannot even change her hair colour without permission. The newsreader is telling us that half of Zaire just got arrested and we wonder why she's wearing that weird blouse.

The eternal youth theory Thinness in girls reaches a peak at about the age of 12, just before the body changes of puberty. Some people think that women who want to remain very thin also do not really want to grow up. Many of the models used to display heavy makeup and low-cut gowns are in fact 12-and 13-year-olds who have not yet been through the body change ingeniously disguised as women. Older women are fearful of age, character lines, hair that gets darker and then turns grey; younger women are afraid of the changes that puberty brings, afraid to grow up, knowing that a pre-pubescent body is the one most glorified.

The theory of learned behaviour

Monkey see, monkey do. Part of the initiation of growing up, part of watching adult women and learning how to be an adult, is learning that we are supposed to dislike our bodies, or at least bits of them. Or at least have one bit that you don't like (pick a part, any part). A *Glamour* magazine survey of 33,000 of its readers revealed that only 13 percent of respondents thought that their mothers were satisfied with their bodies. (Fathers were not considered.)

> I think most girls and ladies think they are the wrong shape and are fat because these days it's supposedly in to be very thin. It's put across in magazines, TV, all media to look like the small percent of people who model. I think to fix this problem magazines, TV, etc. should have more "normal"-sized models modelling.
>
> Naomi, 12

The control theory

Fat people are most often wrongly seen to have "let themselves go." In a world where they do not have very much power, some people take pride in conquering their body's natural needs and being in "control." Seeming to be in control is seen to be a virtue. This is why people talk of punishing themselves with exercise or with guilt for performing a natural function such as being hungry and eating. "I can't control my life but I can control my eating" is a common feeling of someone with an eating disorder. (Unfortunately this really translates to, "I can't control my life but I sure as hell can control getting more miserable and unhealthy.")

The war on the body theory

The natural body is seen as the enemy. *Utne Reader* magazine put it this way: "We have declared war on our bodies...our overworked, high-speed lifestyles have severed any relationship between our bodies and the cycles of nature, including the body's own natural rhythms." This is part of the reason plastic surgeons think they can get away with saying small breasts are "deformed." Technology is always good and any invention should be tried out, but the natural body is bad, defective, primitive, must be made to submit to drugs, obsessive dieting, being cut open, and having foreign bodies inserted.

The femininity theory Old-fashioned notions of "femininity" suggested that a woman should not eat well, but "like a bird," be fragile, quiet (squeaky, even), modest, powerless, supportive, and retiring—in short "ladylike." She should make and serve food for others but hold back on eating herself. This lack of appetite is often seen to apply to other wants such as ambition, self-fulfilment, and personal pursuits.

The brainwash theory Fashion arbiters, magazine editors, and beauty and fashion writers are all participating in the relentless brainwashing that thin is good. The designers only provide samples in size 8. Feeling guilty about this, and doing what they can to redress the balance, the magazines try to run positive stories about self-esteem and body image, and end up with a confusing collage of opposing messages.

The capitalism theory The trend to more and more thinness as an ideal has coincided with the rise of women as an economically powerful group. There are more young, single women delaying marriage and childbirth or rejecting both options altogether, with "disposable income" to spend on themselves. There is extra money to be made from such women, as well as from women who can be made to feel that they are "losing their looks" through drudgery and age. The easiest way to sell people something is to convince them they need it: so the campaigns denigrate the most common shape of women as unsightly or unwanted. Not much money can be made by telling women there isn't anything wrong with them and they don't need to buy anything to fix it. The "You're too fat" message is marketing, not fact.

The duty theory It is a duty for women to "make the best of themselves," to show men that they want their approval. Submitting to this is supposed to be part of a woman's lot. This theory is encouraged by those who sell cosmetics and want you to pay $70 to be wrapped in some plankton and Saran Wrap as a useless cellulite "treatment."

Probably a mix of many or all of these theories contributes to the imposed thin ideal. (Also it may have something to do with aliens and strange circles in wheat fields. This would be part of the Gullible Loony Theory.)

How do you judge your size and shape?

Cartoonist Nicole Hollander says: "My weight is perfect for my height, which varies."

According to Dr. Peter Clark, head of a Sydney hospital eating-disorders clinic, "Any weight you feel comfortable with is the right weight. Things like the pinch test are a load of garbage."

Body-mass index The body-mass index is one way of assessing weight but is not a suitable test for anyone less than 18 years old.

In 1990 the Australian Bureau of Statistics National Health Survey concluded that 48 percent of both men and women were of an acceptable body weight judged on the body-mass index (BMI) scale. The way you find your BMI is to get your calculator, or your brain if you're a math whiz, find your weight in kilograms and your height in metres squared. Now divide your *weight* by your *height squared*. For example, if you weigh 52 kilos and your height is 1.58 metres, squared it's 2.4964. You divide 2.4964 into 52 and get 20.8299. That answer, 20.8, is your body-mass index.

Underweight is defined as a BMI of less than 20, acceptable as 20 to 25, overweight as 26 to 30, and obese as more than 30. According to the Bureau, women were less likely than men to be overweight and more likely to be underweight. (This formula only works using metric measures—kilograms and metres. You can find out what you weigh in kilos if you divide your weight in pounds by 2.2. To calculate your height in metres, divide inches by 39.37.)

Most young women (18 to 24 years) who were not at an acceptable weight were underweight. Nearly one-third of young women were underweight, only 8.1 percent were overweight, and only 2.8 percent were obese. Yet people in this age group were more likely to diet than others.

Some doctors say that "overweight" is defined as a BMI in the top 15 percent of the population, no matter what the score is. The big problem with the body-mass index is that it ignores where the fat is on the body, the fact that muscle weighs more than fat, and genes.

> At 30, I am 210 pounds, most of which is muscle, but certainly not all. I come from large-boned European ancestors and consider myself to be fairly strong and healthy-looking. Men don't seem to have been put off by my non-stereotype body—I've had a fair few long-term relationships, sexual flings, and offers. I must say the one thing about not being a "10" is that the guys you get with (the serious ones) are attracted by you as a person right from the start, not superficial attraction fuelled by magazine hype.
>
> Anne

The waist-hip ratio A better measure of whether your shape is healthy is the amount of flesh around your waist compared to your hips. If you have been through puberty and your waist is bigger than your hips, you may be in need of some exercise. (Or you may be five months pregnant, I can't tell from here.) If your waist is smaller than your hips you most likely have no problems.

To get your waist-hip ratio (WHR) you divide your waist circumference by your hip circumference. For example, if your waist is 75 centimetres and your hips are 97 centimetres your WHR is 0.77. In young children a WHR of 1.1 is common, going down to 0.8 for many young women after puberty. (Calculate your measurements in centimetres by multiplying inches by 2.54. For example, if your waist is 28 inches it is 71 centimetres, and if your hips are 35 inches they're 89 centimetres, which gives you a waist-hip ratio of 0.80 if you round off all the numbers. Easy, isn't it?)

The waist-hip ratio is used to determine people at greater risk of heart disease later in life: this is where the "beer belly" (waist bigger than hips) really shows up as dangerous. In other words, hips are good for you, "beer bellies" bad.

🙎

Weight-for-height charts Ignore most of the weight-for-height charts you see in doctors' offices and in government publications. Some of them have been reprinted from tables put together decades ago and are no longer considered relevant or accurate. The more specific a chart is, the less useful it is.

The weight-for-height charts do not take into account that muscle weighs more than fat; that everyone weighs more as they get older, once they have stopped growing, or if there is water retention due to hormonal cycles; and that the definitions of acceptable weight can change. One researcher at the National Institute on Aging says the charts are relevant only for people in their early forties.

Weight-for-height charts should include a range of healthy weights—for example, from 100 pounds to 124 pounds—not an individual number such as 110 pounds. This allows for the wide diversity of human beings who are all different and don't always fit neatly onto charts and into statistics. Not to mention their trousers.

🙎

Body fat percentage Women need about 17 percent of their body weight as fat in order to menstruate and about 22 percent fat in order to have regular menstrual cycles. Below 20 percent is the average at which women stop having periods.

Doctors involved in athletics accept 14 to 20 percent body fat on women. The *Beauty Myth* by Naomi Wolf says that from birth girls have 10 to 15 percent more fat than boys. The average healthy 20-year-old female has 28.7 percent body fat. By middle age, women cross-culturally have about 38 percent body fat.

Wondering why those shop dummies have such thin hips? They haven't started menstruating (what a thought). No, really, a study of shop mannequins has shown they have been getting thinner since the 1950s, and the modern ones, if they were real women, would not have enough body fat on them to menstruate.

The right size and shape for you If you eat healthy food and have a few indulgences every now and again and if you also exercise three times a week for more than half an hour, you are at the size and shape you should be. This formula is agreed upon by doctors, nutritionists, and body-image consultants. If anybody tells you any different, they're either misled or trying to sell you something. You may shout at them.

Further reading

Boston Women's Health Book Collective, *The New Our Bodies Ourselves* (updated edition; New York: Touchstone Books, 1992). A fantastic reference, a huge soft-cover book all about the natural female body, how it works, what it looks like, common ailments and what to do about them.

Edward Shorter, *A History of Women's Bodies* (New York: Basic Books, 1982).

Dr. Dale Atrens, *Don't Diet* (New York: Bantam, 1988).

Naomi Wolf, *The Beauty Myth* (New York: William Morrow, 1991).

Susan Faludi, *Backlash; The Undeclared War against Women* (New York: Crown, 1991),

Shelley Povey, *Being Fat Is Not a Sin* (London: Pandora, 1989).

chapter two

Weight for me

Food

Food as a sin "Oh, I mustn't," "Oh, I really shouldn't," "It will go straight to my hips." I guess we're just not encouraged to say, "Oh, no, I couldn't possibly. It would go straight to the production of skin cells, my central nervous system, and my toenail growth." (Normal body functioning accounts for 70 percent of daily energy expenditure.)

British *Slimmer* magazine has a "Shapescope" astrology column which in one month tells Aquarians that they have a body like an intricate machine and should not neglect their health (as if) and Scorpios they are going to meet someone new so they'd better lose weight. Pisces must say "no" to temptation in October. In fact there is an awful lot about temptation: Librans should only have romance as a temptation if they lose weight; Aries need willpower; Geminis need determination *and* willpower (they're not eating for two, after all); and Leos shouldn't be giving in to tasty tidbits. Virgos, too, must not give in to temptation.

Australian *Cleo* magazine's survey "Love, Sex and the Dieting Woman" found that 67 percent of women feel guilty every day about eating.

According to diet lore, "indulging" or "giving in to temptation" is a "sin." (Strangling a few people is a sin. Invading East Timor is a sin. "Ethnic cleansing" is a sin. Testing nuclear weapons in the Pacific is a sin. I'm sorry, but eating doesn't quite make the grade.)

Australian *Who Weekly* magazine, which has run many stories about eating disorders, kicked off 1994 with its front-cover screamer "Diet Winners and Sinners of the Year: Here's the Scoop on Who Got Fat, Who Got Fit and How They Did It."

English comedian Jennifer Saunders says, "I'm completely neurotic about [weight]. I've always been overweight. Actually I haven't always been overweight. I started as soon as I became this moody sort of schoolgirl...I put on weight and then dieted at school. Cup of soup for lunch and then you'd go across to the shop and buy six Mars Bars. No-one's teaching you anything: you should just eat normally. Just be sane about it. Not like these neurotic people who go, 'Well, that's a bit naughty isn't it, what you're eating?' Naughty! I'm eating! It's food. I'm EATING IT!...I KNOW I'M BEING NAUGHTY. EATING FOOD IS WRONG ALTOGETHER."

> If I'm out to dinner and everyone orders a dessert, I order one too. What I've learned to do is just take two bites and push the plate away. After all, you don't have to eat everything on your plate. Normally my husband finishes it off!
>
> Cindy Crawford, model

Seven thousand respondents to a *Mirabella* magazine survey revealed that those who were extremely overweight ate the most candy but, at 47 percent, the dangerously *underweight* ate more cakes and cookies than anyone else. The most craved foods were chocolate and ice cream. Chocolate is seen as the biggest sin and so consequently it is the biggest craving.

The gender gap: show us your portion Traditionally food is served in its best and largest proportions to the men: as a reward for status, as fuel for hunting. Biscuits, like handkerchiefs, come in "man size." Little children in countries where there is not enough food will have more chance of survival if they are boys:

food is not the devil : proof

← quite pointy

FIG 1: BEELZEBUB

FIG 2: THE MUSHROOM

they are given more food. Having a smaller portion used to be seen as ladylike, dainty, mysterious. Fanatical Christian girls were praised in years gone by for refusing to eat, fainting, and having hallucinations (visions from the Lord). Their wasted bodies were seen as proof that they could live on faith alone. To be thin and deprived was to be "good."

Food as a reward Eating is often associated with reward in our society—an ice cream for being good, candies after eating our "greens," a celebratory meal, a birthday cake. Food gets mixed up with love or with comfort and security for some people. Cooking is often an act of love and nourishment from a parent or lover and it becomes symbolic of being cared for and protected.

SUGAR HIT

The smell or appearance of food "induces an anticipatory increase in insulin (blood sugar), and in appetite," say Peter Dally and Joan Gomez, authors of *Understanding Anorexia and Obesity.* "The pleasurable feelings associated with the beginning of a meal are due to endorphins, self-made opiates which give a sense of well-being. For most people the endorphin concentration falls away quickly as the meal progresses."

> I read an article by a leading women's nutritionist which said that any guilt feelings about eating certain types of foods could be described as an eating disorder. Well, that's me to a T! A bundle of guilt feelings. I love chocolate more than any other food (except maybe tortellini) and I have convinced myself that this is the source of all my problems. I have tried everything to cut down on the choccy habit—the latest is to add up the money I've saved from resisting temptation and buy something as a reward. This seems to make it even harder to resist and I get into a terrible tizz about it all and if I break down and eat some chocolate I feel so bad about myself.
>
> Margaret

Food pornography

The glossy, full-colour pictures of chocolate cakes and fruit custard flans in magazines that also carry diets are a forbidden realm but an irresistible one. One ice cream is described in sexual advertising as "wicked." Another is "to die for." Denial of food is strongly linked to an obsession with it. Some anorexics and bulimics throw elaborate dinner parties, worship food, become "foodies." They cannot eat it or absorb it but they must be near it. It's a kind of masochistic torture.

Food obsession Most diet books encourage the food obsession. Margaret O'Sullivan's *The Heavenly Body Diet* suggests that women keep a "food diary."

"It's absolutely essential," she said while promoting her book. "It takes me no more than three minutes and I do it in bed at night or during the commercial breaks when I'm watching television."

> I eat normally for a few months until I find the enthusiasm or mental strength to starve myself again. I find it really difficult as I love my food too much and I can't bear to miss out on it for too long.
>
> Louise, 19

She, too, talks of "keeping your weight under control" by counting calories weekly rather than daily. This she sees as an incredible freedom! "If you indulge every now and again you simply take extra care on the other days." This hardly revolutionary idea, along with its boring calorie-counting obsession, was promoted on almost a full page of a Sydney newspaper.

Maybe it started with that weirdo Bible story. I mean, a woman eats an apple—one little apple! And the next thing you know everyone's chucked out of the Garden of Eden and all the evils of the earth, including lawyers and public transport ticket inspectors, famine and pestilence, are visited upon the earth by a vengeful and furious all-powerful God. No wonder women feel guilty about eating. Thankfully Eve wasn't offered a piece of black forest cake by that old snakie thing or we'd all be pulverised into atoms.

> I began losing weight. I was 123 pounds in ninth grade and by the time eleventh grade began I was 90 pounds and everyone told me how good I looked. I lost interest in food. My eating habits are still appalling. Today I've had a donut, Hershey's Kisses, pizza, Coke, and three oranges. I really worry about my kids adopting my eating habits.
>
> Kim, 24

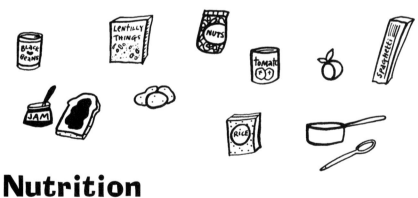

Nutrition

Healthy eating In 1994 the top-selling products at American supermarkets were carbonated drinks, candy, soups, chips, and snacks. I hope you were not expecting them to be unprocessed bran, kelp by-products, and agar-agar. No, Americans are more your sort of Cocoa Puffs nutritionists. Together, we eat almost 22 billion fast-food meals a year.

So, if we assume that we should not be drinking 8 quarts of Coke and having a lardburger every couple of hours, how *should* we be eating?

The Victorian Health Promotion Foundation's Eating Behavior Project suggests some ideas for healthier eating:

- Give yourself permission to eat.
- "Legalise" all foods without feeling guilt.
- Avoid counting calories.
- Use hunger as the cue for eating, not the time of day or habit.
- Eat small meals about every three to five hours.
- Trust your food choices—eat anything you want, forbid nothing.
- Sit down while eating.
- Don't hide away and eat alone—create a pleasant environment and table to eat at.
- Focus your senses on food, its colour, smell, texture, and taste. (They also mention sounds, but if your food is singing, put it away.)
- Notice how your body reacts to certain foods.

There are not many rules for healthy eating, but here they are:

- Don't diet: ever.
- Eat what your body wants you to.
- Vary your food so you don't get bored.
- Don't stick popcorn up your nose.
- Don't trust food advertising.
- Know where your food comes from.
- Don't use added salt.
- Eat fresh food whenever possible.
- Eat as much organically produced food as you can afford.
- If you get into a food fight, make sure you have the custard.

The food groups Forget the old four food groups you learned years ago—they have been modified. Modified, hell, nutrition's a completely different beastie.

Don't take any notice of the magazine that said, "Peruse your plate and leave something on it. There's no reason to eat all the food you're served just because it's there. Your main course arrives with chicken, roast pumpkin and green beans. Eat two of the three choices and leave the third one after a little taste." Nooooooooooo! Eat some of all three!

Your body needs regular hits of the following things: water; vitamins A, C, D, E, K, and B complex; calcium; iron; folic acid; magnesium; iron; zinc; phosphorus; potassium; sodium (no need to add it, it's in most foods already); sulphur; iodine; complex carbohydrates; protein; essential fatty acids; and fibre. The key is in eating a *variety* of foods to get all the goodies.

> How could anorexia be so bad? Once I lose the weight I want, I'll keep going so if I pig out I don't gain fat, I gain weight. Then I'll be able to stop—I can't go without food for long, think of all the white chocolate and glazed donuts!
>
> Summer

Generally, we tend to have too much fat, alcohol, sugar, salt, and animal protein and not enough green leafy things, vegetables, fruit, bread, and grains.

Daily needs

Meats and meat alternatives—including fish, the odd egg, nuts, seeds—once a day (go easy on the salami!), twice for a woman who is pregnant, for extra iron, zinc, and protein.

Milk and dairy products—including cheese and yoghurt—2 serves (this could be a glass of milk and a small tub of yoghurt). Pregnant women need 3 serves for extra protein and calcium.

Veggies—you know, the stuff at the vegetable market. Go wild and eat lots but have at least 4 serves of different veggies a day. Lentils and legumes are included here.

Fruit—"An apple a day..." Fresh is best—three different types a day.

Breads and cereal—important for fibre. Include rice and pasta. Go for it with 5 and preferably more serves a day. (Not so difficult when a serve is a slice of bread or half a cup of cereal.) Pregnant and active women may need 7 to 8 serves a day. Very active adults and growing teenagers can need up to 9 to 12 serves a day (preferably wholemeal).

And remember, a cakie a day keeps the madness away. This is a loose guide only: you don't want to be weighing bits of food and counting up slices and generally getting obsessed with it. Food is not mathematics. Life is too short to weigh lentils.

I like this idea the best: Many nutritionists just divide the food groups into three sections: eat less fat, oil, and sugar; eat moderate amounts of meat, fish, poultry, eggs, and dairy foods; and eat lots of fruit, vegetables, legumes, bread, and cereals. How simple is that?

You'll find that this is probably what your body is asking for once it settles down anyway. You'll be lying there and your body will say, "I'd like some spinach and something kind of crunchy, maybe in a more lurid shade of orange." "A carrot?" you'll inquire. "That's it," the body will say. "I'll have a couple of those carroty things and something red and round and deliciously squishy that explodes in your mouth." "I believe that's what they refer to in intellectual circles as a cherry tomato," you'll reply. "And I want a cheese sandwich and a Junior Mint. Later I may toy with leeks."

If somebody hassles you about eating too much, or eating between meals, strike them repeatedly with this book.

Osteoporosis This is a deficiency disease. The bones lose minerals, particularly calcium, and become brittle and weak, often causing stooping and breaking bones in old age. The decline in bone strength tends to speed up after menopause. Technically, the term refers to people who have lost 50 to 75 percent of their original bone material. Although generally we are told, especially by dairy organisations, that dairy-food calcium intake is the key to protecting ourselves, excessive animal protein consumption, including milk consumption, has been linked to osteoporosis.

The average measurable bone loss in a woman meat-eater at 65 years old in America is 35 percent. The average rate for her vegetarian sister at the same age: 7 percent. It seems that the more animal protein we eat (including that from fish), the more calcium our bodies lose.

Unchallenged research shows that even very high calcium intakes are cancelled out by high animal protein consumption. Bantu women have a dangerously low calcium intake by our standards, but they eat virtually no ani-

> I used food to make me feel better when I was in a state of discomfort. I am now in my healthy weight range and I have worked hard to break the relationship with food and comfort. Now food is for nutrition.
>
> Millie, 24

mal protein. Their osteoporosis rate is very low. This doesn't mean we should stop taking in calcium: we still need it. But it would seem that rather than simply eating more dairy products, we should be eating less protein supplied by meat.

Physical activity from a young age is also linked to low rates of osteoporosis, so get dancing.

Further information

To know more in detail about which foods have which goodies, ring your regional or state health department and get them to send you some nutritional information. A visit to a dietician or a good book on different foods might also be useful. Be careful where your books or pamphlets come from. Industry organisations will be very biased in favour of their own products.

> The National Center for Nutrition and Dietetics
> 216 West Jackson Boulevard
> Suite 800
> Chicago, IL 60606
> Phone: (312)899-0040

They can send you pamphlets and books and answer your questions (although you're not supposed to ask about baseball scores).

Most public hospitals and women's health centres employ nutritionists you can go to see.

Further reading

Dr. Phyllis Butow, Jillian Ball, and Fiona Place, *When Eating Is Everything: How to Overcome Your Eating Problems and Change Your Life* (New York: Doubleday, 1991).

Jane Brody, *Jane Brody's Nutrition Book: A Lifetime Guide to Eating Better for Better Health and Weight Control* (New York: Ballantine, 1987).

John Robbins, *Diet for a New America: How Your Food Choices Affect Your Health, Happiness and the Future of Life on Earth* ▶

(N.H.: Stillpoint, 1987). A brilliant book about what we eat and how it is produced, and a healthier and saner way to eat for ourselves and the planet. (For instance, 64 per ent of U.S. cropland is used to grow animal feed: only 2 percent is for fruits and vegetables.)

Jane Brody and Judith E. Brown, *Everywoman's Guide to Nutrition* (Minneapolis: University of Minnesota Press, 1990).

Carlton Fredericks, *The Columbia Encyclopedia of Women's Nutrition* (New York: Putnam, 1989).

Gary Null, *The Vegetarian Handbook* (New York: St. Martin's Press, 1987).

Dieting

On a diet? America is full of girls and women eating only fruit until midday, following diets that claim to shed weight from the hips, thighs, and left earlobe only, chatting with a fake smile to cover the growling of their stomachs. They are looking wistfully at packets of chocolate-chip cookies, eating crispbread that tastes like boiled cardboard, counting up calories, feeling desperate and miserable, and wondering why they're insanely hungry. They are on a diet and it won't work.

> I want to be 103 pounds. I would be happy at 103 pounds.
>
> Marla, 20

Up to 30 percent of American women are on diets at any one time. Many are depriving themselves of almost all the 1,900 calories of energy needed each day to maintain the body functions of a healthy woman. Even those depriving themselves of "eating between meals" are missing out on the essential supply of the 1,900 calories spread across their waking hours.

Why diets make you gain weight I don't mean that diets don't work because you never lose weight but that the weight is almost always regained. Not because you don't have enough willpower but because the body and the mind have special powers to deal with the starvation you are putting yourself through. When you diet, you do lose some weight—not fat, but water and muscle. This dehydration makes you weigh less and look thinner for a little while. Then the body insists you have to eat something. Your mind obsesses with food, it screams out for you to feed yourself. Meanwhile the body reacts by saving fat and storing more every time you eat.

Every time you lose weight, your body goes into coping mode for starvation. Your metabolism slows down so you burn off less fat. The body re-educates itself to work on less food. Valuable muscle tissue, not fat, is eaten away. Food cravings begin, leading to overeating, binge eating, or eating of low-use high-sugar foods such as snack food and chocolate bars. The body stores away more fat, having been programmed now to expect starvation or famine again.

Get this: if you diet, you are actually training your body to become fatter as a protection against further dieting. Your body is an utter smarty-pants.

"The final result is that some women who started off at a good weight-for-height ratio, over a period of 10 or 20 years have steadily increased their weight, size and fat percentage to a point of no return. Obesity, then, can be caused by constant dieting and the fol-

Diet pills: I tried the ones you buy at the chemist at age 15. I lost the few pounds I wanted to, but looking back I really didn't need to lose any weight. I think people need to accept their shape and as this happens they will begin to accept other people's shapes. It would be a boring old world if everyone had the body of an iron man or supermodel.

Teri, 22

lowing weight gain," says community nurse Penelope Goward, who is an expert on body image.

Willpower schmillpower. There is nothing wrong with *you*—there's a lot wrong with dieting. To recover we must listen to our bodies, not work against them, Except in the case of an illness or a disorder, your body knows what it is doing. It has been genetically programmed to do it for thousands of years and no short-term starvation diet can get the better of it.

So what is the secret? The only way is to work with the body, by feeding it healthy food and a few indulgences and exercising as regularly as possible. People who are not obsessed with food, not dieting, not feeling hungry and deprived, accept themselves as they are and live happier lives.

The generally accepted percentage of dieters who regain the weight they have lost is about 95 percent. Dr. Xavier Pi-Sunyer of St. Luke's Hospital in New York says the figure is closer to 85 percent and a 1993 survey by *Consumer Reports* puts it at 75 percent. Other figures of 90 percent and 98 percent have been mentioned but I suspect they may be estimates. The dieting industry certainly doesn't want to publicise the extraordinarily high rate of failure of their programs and potions.

Those who regain the weight they lose do so within two years of their weight-loss programs according to a study by the University of Texas. The study found that when people were taught to eat as they wished, they gained self-confidence and better health (but more on that later).

The body *needs* the extra padding on thighs, hips, and bottoms (where women want to lose it) and will protect itself against starvation. Your body is looking after you, even while you are abusing it. Imagine what it could be like if you worked together.

Dieting makes you sick "Dieting, losing weight and putting it back on again is far worse than maintaining a heavy weight," says Dr. Jane Ogden, author of *Fat Chance!* The stress put on the body by the starvation and sudden eating, and the resultant dramatic changes, is very unhealthy, threatening your immune system and the general workings of your body and its organs. It will also

> I weigh 65 pounds more than I'd like. I have been fat since I was four years old. I have always been a healthy eater. I eat all the right things, not a lot. There was a succession of diets from age four: none worked. I tried calorie-counting diets, magazine diets, doctor diets, acupuncture, laser treatment, prescribed drugs, diet drinks, Gloria Marshall, Nutri-System, Weight Watchers, Jenny Craig. Nothing has worked. So I am still fat.
>
> Melissa, 22

cause stretch marks. The healthy, gradual weight loss that happens on a healthy, abundant diet along with exercise should be no more than two pounds a week.

Dieting makes you depressed

Because dieting doesn't work, people blame a lack of willpower. Dieters blame themselves when they had only a 5 percent chance of success in the first place: less if they had dieted before. By its very nature, dieting makes people unsatisfied, wanting, yearning, unfulfilled. Hunger is depressing. Not being able to enjoy food is depressing. Being terrified of a carrot is so extremely depressing I don't even want to think about it.

Dieting makes you obsessed with food

Penelope Goward explains: "If you lower your calories (as in a diet) the psychical signal your body gets is 'starvation' or 'famine' and responds accordingly. No one can exist on a reduced food intake without exhibiting a 'starvation' response. This over-interest is a normal part of feeling physically hungry every 3 to 5 hours—we instinctively want to feed ourselves. There is increased interest in food which over a period of prolonged dieting can become an induced food obsession—like food fantasies, food dreams, waiting for your next meal, talking about food, planning meals and generally finding food on your mind for most of the time."

useful Bathroom scales

Dieting makes you unhealthy

Dr. Dale Atrens points out in his book *Don't Diet* that the futile pursuit of dieting makes people believe that they cannot lose weight because they haven't the willpower. So they give up attempts to start regular exercise, think they might as well smoke and drink, and eat lots of sugary foods under the mistaken impression that their extra weight necessarily makes them unhealthy. In fact their weight may be perfectly natural and healthy for them.

> I took diet pills. At night I would dream of food, and I stopped taking them and went up to size 14. Then I didn't think about weight gain and started to lose weight. I'm size 10–12 now and I'm quite happy with myself. In Europe now it's okay to be big: big women walk around in bikinis, and no one cares.
>
> Gillian, 19

Penelope Goward says that continued dieting makes your body exhibit signs and symptoms of poor nutrition such as extreme hunger, irritability, depression and anxiety, nervousness, fatigue, listlessness, poor sleep patterns, desire for sugar, and poor concentration. One then finally has to give in to eating, the natural survival instinct.

Dieting makes you stupid

An English study of dieting students showed that they performed much worse than a group of normal eaters when tested on reaction times, rapid information processing, and memory. Doctors believe that part of the problem was the dieters were so obsessed with food and body image they could not concentrate effectively on other tasks. The lack of food was also a shock to the system, causing stress, which reduces concentration and ability to focus. Another explanation would be that diets induce lowered heart rates or starve the brain of glucose. The women who did the least well in the tests were the ones who had been dieting the longest.

Why young people must not diet

Teenagers being hassled by their parents about their eating should show them this

paragraph. *Dieting is dangerous for young people.* Not quite as dangerous as removing your brain and setting fire to it, but pretty close.

These are your growth spurt years. You need the growth, you need the brain power, and you need the energy that good food gives you. You don't need the hassle of dieting. Overweight young people need good food and exercise. But are you really overweight? If you are eating good food and exercising for at least half an hour three times a week (even walking) then your body will be at the right size and shape.

> So what's the diet? Well you eat a hard-boiled egg before every meal and the hard-boiled egg actually eats some of that meal for you.
>
> Comedian Victoria Wood

Here's another thing to show the naggers. *You should be eating between meals.* Well, hurrah! Some soy milk, some sunflower seeds, yoghurt, fruit, vegetables, or a whole-grain cheese-and-lettuce sandwich when you get home from school and something mid-morning are fine. They will help stave off the craving for junk food, like chips and chocolate, very dangerous for teenagers because they're so easy to buy and so unhealthy for you, with all the added fat, sugar, and salt.

A recent national survey revealed that 60 percent of fourth- grade girls were dieting.

But Jenny O'Dea, a Sydney dietician, says dieting is not the answer. "Dieting in growing adolescents impairs growth and restricts nutrients such as protein, iron, calcium and zinc, which teenagers need a lot of. You don't want children and teenagers to be losing weight unless they are very obese. It is normal for them to gain height and weight. Parents also need to realise that it's normal for girls to put on a large percentage of fat. A lot of parents say, 'She's getting fat,' but really she's just getting a womanly shape."

Parents can also help by reassuring teenagers that they do not look like enormous Space Porkers from the Planet Zorg but normal-sized human beings who are the target market for magazines and TV shows with pretend young people in pretend makeup with pretend lighting and pretend personalities.

Food and energy Food provides the energy we need for making our body function and renew itself even while we're asleep or watching a video. The energy is measured in calories. Because of their faster metabolism, some people burn energy (or calories) faster than others. Teenagers, children, pregnant women, and naturally larger people generally need more calories.

Calories are calculated from the composition of different foods. For example, a gram of fat gives 9 calories, a gram of alcohol supplies 7 calories, and a gram of carbohydrate or protein provides 4 calories.

Nutritionists agree that a person should eat at least 1,200 calories a day for safe weight loss. Weight-control centres say their programs offer between 960 and 1,200 calories but one nutrition-

> It makes you feel guilty about everything you eat. Seems skinny people just are better than you because they can stay on a diet. Girlfriends have the biggest influence, they are who you compare yourselves to, if they can lose weight and stay thin and you can't you feel lower than them. What I would give to look like a magazine model. Bodywise, your face is your own individuality coming out but everyone's got the same body or can have. I would want Cindy Crawford's body.
>
> Kylie

ist clocked a certain program's diet at 790 a day. Some short-term diets such as fasts and fruit or liquid diets are below starvation levels of calorie intake.

The trouble with counting calories is that it ignores vitamins and minerals and doesn't care whether or not you've had any greens in the last calendar year. It encourages an obsession with tiny bits of food and discourages listening to your body to find out what it is telling you it needs. There are many other considerations in eating apart from simple calorie consumption. How big are you naturally? How much exercise do you do? Do you feel like having a Popsicle?

Diets and who's flogging them The people who sell diets know they don't work. That's why they keep churning out so many "new" ones in magazines. They know people are desperate to lose weight, and they have to sell magazines to them. And if they run the same healthy nutrition and exercise recommendations in every magazine, they might lose gullible readers to another magazine claiming a "revolution" or a "breakthrough." They know that young readers are influenced and want to look like models. Even though the magazines know that is an impossible dream, they will run "supermodel diets."

Every diet that isn't a plan for general nutrition is a fad diet. Sydney dietician Jo Rogers, who worked for 40 years at the Royal Prince Alfred Hospital, on her retirement let fly at fad diets, naming one magazine diet as promoting "nutritional quackery."

A magazine spokeswoman said the diet was only meant to be short term but Rogers was having none of it. "[The] Wonder Diet was close to a starvation diet and it isn't going to teach people anything, because everyone knows if they starve they'll lose weight. [It] claims... to give you a 'kick start' but that's not helpful because it just involves loss of fluid. As soon as you resume normal eating you regain the weight and then people become disappointed in themselves," she told a magazine interviewer.

"In a successful weight-loss program weight loss will be slow. We need to overcome our obsession with weight and make the best of what we are. The plan should be supported by 30 minutes of exercise three times weekly."

I have tried water diets, no-breakfast diets, no-lunch diets, no-dinner diets, no-food diets. But none work! Because I don't have the willpower. There's a lot of food I don't like so I can't take diets out of the magazines.

Sybilla, 17

The interveiwer asked, "If I needed to shed 10 pounds fast to fit into a slinky cocktail dress, what would you suggest?" That's easy. "Buy another dress," replied Rogers.

A medical magazine asked a panel of four nutritionists to evaluate seven diets in women's magazines published in 1993. Only one was approved, the only diet to take account of recommended daily vitamins and minerals and to encourage a healthy long-term eating plan.

Four of the diets recommended in the women's magazines had less than half the required energy for a woman aged 20 to 30, and were low in important vitamins and minerals, especially iron and zinc.

David Roberts, professor of dietetics and nutrition at Newcastle University, said the first day of the magazine diet Rogers trashed would be more like the diarrhoea diet followed by farting for day two, diarrhoea and farting on day three, and constipation on the rice-only day four. Charming. The low-carbohydrate diets would result in the body losing water, muscle tissue, and "pretty well" no fat, according to nutritionist Rosemary Stanton.

The medical magazine concluded, "The panellists

agreed that women's magazines would continue to publish diets that were anti-social, unpalatable, inflexible, nutritionally unbalanced and that did not consider cost, food availability or the person's likes and dislikes." Basically, the short-term diets in magazines are crap.

Perhaps the dumbest diets are the single-food diets, like the many magazine ones, or the Israeli Army Diet (only apples one day, only cheese another), the Beverly Hills Diet, the Grapefruit Diet, the Banana Diet, the Airline Stewardess Diet (I certainly won't be eating any of *them*), the Rice Diet, the Martini Olive Diet, the Great Whacking Gobs of Lard Diet. Sorry, I made that last one up. All right, I made the last two up.

Health propaganda Health organisations, well funded and with a variety of free publications and credibility with the media, are at the forefront of telling people to lose weight and diet. But are they really sensible angels of mercy or just another part of the anti-fat hysteria?

These organisations do recommend a long-term, healthy eating plan, with exercise, but other attitudes they encourage can be a worry.

The Weight Loss Guide published by the Australian National Heart Foundation has some disturbing messages, including the first section: ways of telling if you are overweight. "Take off your clothes and stand in front of a mirror. Can you see extra flesh where it shouldn't be? Do parts of your body wobble too much? The mirror doesn't lie. While in front of the mirror try the pinch test. Pinch a good layer of skin over your tummy. If you can pinch more than an inch you're likely to benefit from losing some body fat." (The pinch test is rubbish.)

The booklet then recommends the waist-hip ratio and a weight-for-height chart. The only really sensible test here is the waist-hip ratio, if health is the concern. As for the rest of it, the Heart Foundation does not say how much wobble is all right. Given that all healthy bodies and super-lean athletes have wobbly bits, it seems unnecessarily alarmist to suggest that wobbling in itself is a problem at all. There's nothing wrong with the odd wobble, darling. Why do you think belly dancing has been around for thousands of years?

Unfortunately, because of weight-loss propaganda, most women look in the mirror and wrongly believe they have weight "where it shouldn't be": on their hips and thighs.

And as for the mirror not lying, we know this to be untrue. The mirror is telling fibs. The body-image distortions previously displayed only by those with eating disorders are now experienced by what may be a vast majority of women. Some studies suggest that 80 percent of women see themselves as larger than they really are.

The first benefit of weight loss suggested by the National Heart Foundation is "You look better." The second, "Feel better about yourself." The third, "Look younger." The fourth, "Can be more active." It is not until the fifth reason that health is even mentioned: "Can lower blood cholesterol, high blood pressure and high blood-glucose levels."

The diet predators Even though they know so few succeed in losing weight permanently or even for a significant period, plenty of people are happy to take your money for their diet books or "programs."

According to a consumer advocacy magazine, which sent out an undercover investigative reporter, some diet companies use hard-sell tactics. Luckily for them, clients are usually so humiliated by their sense of dieting "failure" that they either blame themselves (with some encouragement from popular myths) or are too embarrassed to make a formal complaint.

Jenny Craig's representative treated the inquiring anonymous magazine representative as if she had already joined up, creating a sense of inevitability; at Gloria Marshall, an Australian weight-control chain, a staff member told the reporter that she could have a $150 discount if she paid on the spot (a $150 discount on $560). The Gloria Marshall representative asked the woman to get her husband to ring with his credit-card number.

> I'm 15 years old and have been on crash diets since I was eleven. But I just can't seem to lose much or last on it long. Being on a diet makes me feel empty and bored. When I talk to my parents they think it's easy to lose weight and aren't interested and I end up upset. Nothing like boredom or stress makes me eat. I just can't help it.
>
> Susie, 15

The magazine found that the weight-loss programs had misleading advertising, confusing price systems (especially Nutri-System), and there were obligations to buy the food marketed by the companies.

The Herbalife consultant did not ask for any health details from the customer. The Jenny Craig staff told the undercover reporter she needed to lose weight but she was not overweight by any health guidelines.

In 1993 an Australian newspaper reporter, rated by a well-known nutritionist as only 5 pounds heavier than underweight and only 10 pounds from dangerously underweight, fronted up at several weight-loss centres to check them out. Jenny Craig's representative said she should lose 10 pounds. Gloria Marshall's employee wanted her to take off 14 pounds to be a "beautiful size 6." That would cost $530. Relax and Swim toning salon in Essendon, Victoria, said 7 pounds should go. Only the Life Be In It Health Solutions Centre told her not to bother and strongly advised her not to go anywhere else.

The Consumer Advocacy and Financial Counselling Association of Victoria investigated the weight-control centres in 1992 and concluded that many had unfair policies and 80 percent of the consumers surveyed felt they were not successful either at losing weight or keeping it off as a result of their program. Some spent up to $2,250 each. If we accept that conservative estimate it means that 80 percent of the $375 million a year spent in Australia on weight-loss programs is wasted. (Americans spend a bamboozling $30 billion a year on diet programs and diet products.)

The cigarette diet Millions of women who say they want to lose weight to be healthier smoke cigarettes, afraid to give up in case they put on weight. Even the most furious anti-fat lobbyist has to admit that smoking cigarettes is a much greater danger to your health than extra weight.

Diet drugs make you insane Even recommended doses can cause insomnia, crankiness, and false levels of energy. Former users report addiction, collapses, hallucinations, malnutrition, and the loss of jobs and friends. These pills are "legalised uppers" as one addict wrote in her account to a teen magazine. When she came off them "cold turkey," without help, her heart rate dropped almost enough to kill her.

I'm fat...I'm not overweight for my height but I have stretch marks all over my hips and thighs. I read once in *Dolly* that if you can pinch more than one inch of fat from your thighs, stomach, or underarm, you need toning.* I have tried so many diets. You wouldn't believe how many. Since I turned 15 six months ago I have been on a constant diet. Usually I go for about a fortnight living on virtually nothing (1,000 calories a day) and then I can't stand it any more and so I eat whatever I want. And the worst bit is I'm not losing any weight. If you ask me, it sucks. It is just not fair. My philosophy is that if you've got a good bod, guys will forgive you for being ugly. Boys like girls who are thin.

Sandra

*Note: the pinch test is not a useful guide to anything.

Appetite suppressants are very dangerous because your appetite is a natural thing. Eating when you're not hungry may be a problem but it's not a great idea to suppress your real hunger. The Australian Society for the Study of Obesity has identified an overprescription of drugs and uncovered evidence that sales of some "speed" prescribed as appetite suppressants exceeded the number of prescriptions written. In 1989, 410,000 prescriptions were issued to Australians for appetite suppressants, costing more than $18 million. These prescriptions were written by doctors and I'd like to give them a good slapping.

Other stupid ideas Bulking agents that make you feel full or puff up in your stomach are weird and can be dangerous. Lozenges to deaden taste, sold in pharmacies, can make your tongue and mouth go numb and must be the ultimate in party-pooper ideas, making it impossible to enjoy food. This in turn encourages you to eat more to get the pleasure you once had.

Liquid diets have killed a few people and spectacularly failed others. This rapid weight loss is almost always followed by rapid weight gain, placing a stress on the body much more dangerous than obesity. A teen magazine said that liquid diets do not have a long-term effect, make it harder to lose weight, and the sugar level in drinks makes you crave more sugar and food. *Allure* warned against the juice fasting: some U.S. juice companies were sug-

> When I was 17 years to 19 years old I was trying diet pills (average of ten a day) and laxatives. Diet pills and medications like it should be prescription only.
>
> Annette, 25

gesting a seven-day fast using their products. The National Institutes of Health recommended that no dieter undertake a regime of less than 800 calories a day without medical supervision. The juice diet had 90.

Fasting is also stupid. I don't care what anybody says about toxins or religious experiences.

Hip and thigh diets, or others claiming to work on one part of the body, are just bizarre. I mean, wouldn't you be a teensy bit suspicious of the earlobe diet, or the ankle-and-left-buttock diet? The lose-weight-from-your-knees-and-your-instep diet? "No, I can't have a cakie thing, I'm trying to lose weight from my wrists." Get outta here.

"Replacements" A cookie is not a meal. A small pile of gravel is not a meal. A powdered drink is not a meal. There is almost nothing more than these supplements likely to drive you to eating a real meal or a large buffalo with Mint Milanos very soon afterwards. We don't need to replace meals with something else. We need to replace our diet obsession with meals.

English *Slimmer* magazine says, "The [meal replacement] cookies may be filling (due to their high fibre content) and more nutritious than ordinary biscuits (due to an added vitamin and mineral mix) but they don't re-train your eating habits and they're expensive."

On another page of the same issue of the magazine it says, strangely, "Those curves need keeping in check." Working round to a promotion the magazine continues, "Limmits

> Magazine diets usually involve spending money on foods that we don't normally keep around the house, or spending time exercising daily which I'm too lazy to attempt, so I just stay with the cheap and simple starvation diet. The few pounds I do lose I put straight back on again in a week.
>
> Fran, 19

Meal replacements are a convenient way to control your calorie intake...they can be used to replace one or two meals during the

CUP
'o'
GRUEL

not a meal ...   not a meal ...

not even close ...   get a grip!

day, followed by a healthy balanced meal in the evening...Limmits are high in fibre, which makes them pleasantly filling and satisfying [so is sawdust, presumably], helping you to avoid feeling hungry between meals [or meal replacements?]...We have 100 samples of Limmits Strawberry Cream biscuits to give to *Slimmer* readers who send their name and address..." And their brain?

Why laxatives do not work Laxatives do not make you lose fat because the nutrients are absorbed before the waste is expelled. The only "weight loss" is a temporary loss of water.

Tea time The herbal teas usually associated with weight loss are simple diuretics, which only get rid of water. Magazine ads for Yoland Lim's Oriental Secret go on to reveal that his only secret is having the audacity to claim that his capsules are a seven-day slimming program on which "you can lose pounds in the shortest possible time." The ingredients? Just herbs and vitamins.

The solution There *is* a solution. It means no more hunger, no more expensive foods and supplements you wouldn't normally buy. It does mean you have to be brave and willing to buy fresh food. It means the end of guilt, the end of forbidden foods, the end of food obsession. It means throwing away all the diets and trying to find the time to exercise if you can.

It means *eating whatever you want to*. Aaaaaargh! This is a revolutionary idea and scary for people who crave chocolates and "bad" foods all the time. But think about it—maybe the only reason you're so crazy about those foods is that you won't let yourself have them.

You have to make friends with your body, live in it and trust it.

Dr. Jane Ogden's theory is that if you take away food restrictions and dieting to lose weight, food becomes less of an obsession, you eat when you need to eat, and your body finds its natural weight. "There is no need for most people to expect a large weight increase when they stop dieting—their bodies usually find a natural, set weight," she explains.

Community nurse Penelope Goward agrees: "Stop dieting and restricting food. We need to give ourselves permission to eat and trust our body's signals. Eat when you are hungry (about every three to five hours) and when you want to. Do not add up any calories or think about the nutritional value of food. Rely on and trust your own body."

Long-time American dieters who have followed this idea are at first a little freaked out by all the permission. Geneen Roth, who runs workshops called Breaking Free, says, "They think they will eat 12 gallons of ice cream and six pizzas and dozens of dough-nuts." When she stopped dieting herself, Roth at first ate only choco-late-chip cookies and the dough they were made from. She says she was learning what her body was really asking for. She levelled off after the first gain.

When Lauralee Roark, who now runs Beyond Hunger work-shops, stopped after years of dieting, she said, "It was like letting the tiger out of the cage. I ate everything that wasn't nailed down...[but] now my body says 'broccoli' as loud as it once said 'chocolate.'"

Penelope Goward adds, "Deal with the underlying issues that cause you to eat when you are not hungry. Attend women's groups or compulsive eating and body image workshops that have an anti-diet approach. Stop discussions about weight control, bodies, di-ets and weight, and stop complimenting others for weight loss.

"Most of us are not meant to be thin or even slim by today's standards. We're not all the same weight for the same reason we're not all the same height, or same hair colour, or whatever. Accept and like yourself for who you are. Stop postponing your life until you are an acceptable shape and size. Feel good about yourself, for who you are and your unique contributions to life."

Further reading

Susan Kano, *Making Peace with Food: A Step by Step Guide to Freedom from the Diet Weight Conflicts* (Boston: Amity Publishing, 1985).

Dr. Dale Atrens, *Don't Diet* (New York: Bantam, 1988).

B. Schwartz, *Diets Don't Work* (Houston:Breakthru, 1982).

Obesity

What is obese? Perfectly

normal women will wail about being "fat" or "obese." But what does "obese" mean exactly?

Obesity is defined by some as when a fully developed person is over 30 on the body-mass index scale (see page 18). Others say it is being 20 percent or more above what is considered one's ideal weight range. It is different from being overweight, although the two are often lumped together as if there were no difference.

Who is obese? Obesity

seems to be increasing in American society—probably as a result of less exercise and more junk food and fast food, which have high fat and salt contents. A series of Na-

I eat breakfast because I have to as Mum makes that every morning, and she makes my lunch every day but I never eat that. I always chuck it in a bin at school. My dinner I usually end up flushing down the toilet, I wait until everyone has left the kitchen, and then head for the toilet and lie to Mum and say I've already eaten. I also drink about two quarts of water a day as I heard that water breaks up fat* and makes it easier to lose it. I still get the urge to pig out, say, if I'm depressed and then I end up buying a packet of Twinkies and eat the whole packet. I have reached my goal of being skinnier than my sister. I found out recently that my sister had bulimia.

Julie, 16

*Note: water does not "break up fat."

tional Health and Nutrition Examination Surveys found that 33.4 percent of adults were overweight or obese in 1988–91, 8 percent more than in 1976–80.

One easy way to become obese is to go on a lot of diets. (Sounds crazy? The diet section explains.)

A psychologist from a Sydney eating-disorders clinic says the clinic found large differences between obese men and women. Men tended to be larger, not worried about their weight, and found it easier to lose the weight. Women had a more complex attitude to food—many expected to cook for others but remain slim.

Causes of obesity The most common cause of obesity is overeating and lack of exercise, sometimes for psychological reasons. (Just as undereating, overtalking, and underpoliteness and everything else we do are caused by psychological reasons.) "We live in a society that says fat is bad," says community health nurse Penelope Goward. "People panic and start getting obsessed about it and they end up eating more. If we didn't live in a society which suffers from fat phobia, we wouldn't have so many fat people." She believes many fat people have a good self-image and that those who don't, have a bad one imposed by the disapproval of others.

Starting young A children's hospital dietician, Susan Thompson, says, "If a child has two obese parents he or she has an 80 percent chance of being obese. Children with two slim parents have a less than 10 per cent chance of being obese. Quite a lot of studies have shown that obesity is genetic rather than environmental...[but] the biggest contributing factors would be a high fat intake, overeating and a lack of activity. Children's activity levels are dropping." Kids who exercise about as much as a housebrick are at the highest risk.

A quarter of all American students between the ages of 6 and 17 are overweight, according to recent studies. In Australia, Dr. John Court, director of Melbourne's Centre for Adolescent Health, told a national conference on children's nutrition that parents and teachers should not pressure "fat" children to lose weight. Genetics made up some of the reasons and lack of exercise was the main problem, he said. "If you are overweight and that is your constitution then it is not necessarily a health hazard," Dr. Court added. "Parents must recognise the fact that many overweight children are perfectly normal and should not be constantly subjected to diets that set them up for failure."

Is it dangerous? Some doctors say obesity is dangerous; others disagree. As far as I can make out over the din of experts fighting about it, being very, very overweight—obese—does carry some health risks. But it also protects from other risks. Being overweight or slightly overweight usually does not carry increased risk of health problems. That is, you can carry around a few extra pounds above your healthy weight range without increasing your risk of anything much except carrying around extra weight.

Anyway, here are the arguments: many cardiologists, who do not like obesity at all, say obese people are twice as likely to die early as people in a "healthy" weight range, and more likely to contract disease, have accidents, and commit suicide. Other studies find that obese people are less likely to fall ill than the underweight (see diet section, page 33).

It is definitely possible to be fat and healthy. A "spare tyre" around the middle is dangerous but evenly distributed fat is not necessarily dangerous and, in fact, may mean fewer health problems than for the underweight.

Real obesity can cause health problems, including diabetes and heart disease. It can be very difficult for obese people to lose weight, partly because of habit and partly because their metabolisms can be very slow. Ironically, some obese people are prone to malnutrition because they eat junk food and do not get enough vitamins and minerals. But obese people do not necessarily eat more than thin people.

Penelope Goward, community health nurse and the head of the Victorian Health Promotion Foundation's Body Image and Eating Behaviour Project (who must have a very large business card), says, "Obese people need to be assessed with respect. Not all of them

have underlying problems. Sometimes it's just good old genetics and their bodies are adapted to that size. If there are underlying [psychological] issues, they can be worked on." She recommends that people who think they have a problem with obesity should contact a community health nurse, doctor, or counsellor.

Eating disorders

Who has eating disorders? "Almost all women do have an eating disorder," says Dr. Peter Clark from the eating-disorders clinic at a Sydney hospital. "All the magazines emphasise it and even a book like this will draw attention to it again...if it were a book for men it would only have one paragraph. Eating disorders are increasing in men but not as much as they are in women."

And now for the statistics. The National Association of Anorexia Nervosa and Associated Disorders has reported that the number of eating disorders has reached epidemic levels. According to another eating-disorders organisation, the post-1960 girl sees more images of impossibly "beautiful" women in "sexy" poses in one day than her mother saw through her entire adolescence.

Statistics from the National Association of Anorexia Nervosa and Associated Disorders show that 7 million American women and 1 million men suffer from anorexia or bulimia. Both eating disorders are most prevalent in young women. The problems usually begin in the teenage years. In 10 percent of cases, the illness begins at 10 years old or younger.

Many teenage girls use extreme dieting ideas to try to lose weight. A study of 600 adolescent boys and girls at La Trobe University in Australia found that extreme weight-loss methods associated with anorexia and bulimia had been tried by 48 percent of girls and 26 percent of boys: at least weekly by 13 percent of girls and 9 percent of boys.

A study of 30 bulimic and 30 anorexic patients at a Sydney clinic found that they shared many things, including a dissatisfaction with their thighs and stomachs. Eighty-three percent of the bulimic patients vomited each week (an average of 11.7

times), 33 percent abused laxatives, 10 percent took diet pills. About one-quarter of the anorexics made themselves vomit on average four times a week.

The mean age at which both groups started worrying about their weight was about 14 years 7 months. About 15 years 7 months was the mean age for the onset of dieting and disordered eating behaviour. Thirteen percent of the bulimics had a history of anorexia, and 46 percent of the anorexics displayed features of bulimia. Sixty percent of anorexics weighed themselves at least several times a week, but 30 percent rarely or never did. Fifty to 60 percent of both groups did not count calories. Only 46 percent of the anorexia patients admitted they were too thin.

That's a lot of numbers adding up to a lot of sadness.

Most of the definitions and symptoms of anorexia and bulimia presented here are culled from information provided by the eating-disorders clinic, as well as government health information, and books. Not all people with eating disorders are the same, so the symptoms and feelings described are best viewed as tendencies rather than rules.

Anorexia and bulimia can result in a lifetime struggle with the condition, or even death. Long-term emotional problems are believed to be both cause and effect of the disorders, although sufferers and doctors all agree that the social pressures to diet and to be slender can trigger or encourage the conditions. Many people with anorexia and bulimia have in common a low self-esteem and a cruel perfectionism that allow them no flaws in appearance or performance of any activity undertaken. A small flaw—a wrong note in a whole concert, a 98 percent score—is seen as a failure. "A significant number of anorexics and bulimics have been victims of rape, molestation and incest," according to the clinic. Often their families are having problems, sometimes hidden and not admitted to, but many

—I have binged for three years. I hate it. I hate me. I feel worthless and out of control.—Good luck.

—For ladies with eating problems: stop watching TV and reading glossy glamour magazines—re-educate the mind and the peace with your body will follow.

Graffiti in Queensland University law faculty women's toilets people with eating disorders come from loving families that are healthy and supportive.

Many women with eating disorders are in pursuit of happiness which they believe will come if they look thinner.

Anorexia nervosa The girl in the coffee shop having "lunch" with her friends orders only a glass of water. Her elbows are painfully large compared with her bone-thin arms. Her eyes are shadowed, her hair dull. She says she is not hungry. She is starving.

Anorexia nervosa is a psychological disease that causes a patient to restrict food drastically or not to eat food at all. It is carelessly called a "slimmer's disease"; actually, it is self-imposed starvation to lose weight. Classic anorexics believe they are heading towards the mythical perfect body as demanded by society, and they believe that by controlling their bodies they are controlling their lives.

The National Association of Anorexia Nervosa and Associated Disorders, which offers free counselling, treatment, and support groups, does not keep separate figures on anorexia and bulimia or binge eating and purging because all result from the same "irrational fear of being fat."

For many people, anorexia or another eating disorder is a long-term problem. About 86 percent become anorexic by the age of 20. While 30 percent recover within 5 years, 16 percent continue to suffer for between 11 and 15 years. Only 50 percent are ever fully "cured." And it is estimated that 6 percent of serious cases die, usually from cardiac arrest, failure of their liver, kidneys, or another organ, or from suicide.

Anorexics may have abnormal neatness and control about themselves and their environment, and are perfectionists in every project. Their realities tend to be in extremes. Something is either fabulously good or disgusting, beautiful or ugly, fat or thin. Anorexics, and sometimes their families, may deny any problem and resent offers of help.

Classic anorexics often feel that what they think, say, and do have little or no impact on other people. Control over their bodies substitutes for control over other parts of their lives. Potential anorexics and bulimics tend to be the "good children" who please their parents, who presume this means there is nothing wrong with their children. Anorexics are often passive, agreeable children who do not express their own wants and needs and who can eventually rebel by not eating, creating the first major power struggle in the relationship.

Symptoms can include overexercise, vomiting, laxative abuse, diuretics, appetite suppressants, deceitful behaviour to avoid eating ("I ate before"; "I've had lunch"; "I'm not hungry"), a relentless pursuit of thinness, covering up the body with baggy clothes, a failure to register what the body really looks like (saying "I'm fat" when skeletal), and an obsession with food, shape, and size in oneself and others. Anorexics often memorise calorie charts, read nutritional books, shop for food, and plan elaborate meals they do not eat.

Physical consequences can include loss of periods, weakness, osteoporosis or bone damage, hair loss, pigment changes, skeletal appearance, stunted growth, about a trillion vitamin and mineral deficiencies, starvation, hallucinations, and ultimately, for some, death.

> After six months of throwing up I looked terrible, blisters on my knuckles from rubbing against my teeth, broken capillaries around my eyes, and swollen glands around my jaw. My skin had broken out in spots and most importantly I was experiencing mood swings and bouts of deep depression. I know the only way out of this is to accept my body at its natural weight. But the trouble is I just can't, and I can't see any way out of this. I just don't know how to relate to food any more. I miss being normal, I envy people who eat and enjoy their food. I live for the day the fuller figure comes back into fashion.
>
> Carrie, 23

According to Sydney eating-disorders expert Dr. Clark, the best way to help or cure anorexia is to get early recognition and diagnosis of the problem and early intervention. People who have the onset later in life often have a better chance of recovery. Support from friends or family is another crucial factor. A person who has displayed anorexic behaviour for 20 years has less chance of recovery.

"Often these patients have other problems such as a dysfunctional family. Most remember the time they began worrying about their weight. A brother might say she has a big bum: [this] is a common one," says Dr. Clark. Karen Carpenter, the singer who

I've had anorexia for about 18 months. Eating disorders are almost always the symptom of a very severe emotional problem, *not* a diet gone wrong. Now I realise that starvation was the only way I felt able to communicate the emotional turmoil inside. I was taken to the cardiac ward...I kept telling them there'd been a mistake there was nothing wrong with me. Mum left in hysterics and I was alone in a strange hospital bed while nurses tried to coax me into eating.

In the middle of the night I was woken by a loud alarm. My heart rate had dropped below 35 beats per minute and technically I was dying. I was transferred to the eating-disorders ward at a private hospital. After my repeated refusals to co-operate I was placed on the dreaded "program."

Everything was taken away from me and I was forced to stay in bed in my PJs. I had no visitors, no books, no phone calls. I had to earn my privileges by weight gain. These attempts to pacify my strong will failed and three weeks later I was transferred again to a medical hospital.

This time it was a real emergency: I was taken in an ambulance complete with oxygen mask and stretcher to the intensive care unit. My spirit was cracked by the private hospital's harsh punishments. I left even more absorbed with food and self-hatred than when I arrived. Since then I have had four hospital admissions and still remain at a very low weight. If what I have said so far is any use to you then it is worth the pain of reflecting on it.

Jane, 16

died from anorexia, started dieting when a newspaper article described her as "chubby." Actress Tracey Gold, ironically from the show *Growing Pains*, was hospitalised with anorexia. She started starving herself when a casting agent made a rude comment about her body.

The Sydney clinic adds, "Ambitious, achieving girls between 12 and 25 are especially vulnerable. However, in industrialised countries the condition is becoming epidemic in all age groups and both sexes."

A Perth eating-disorders clinic has reported that girls at private schools have a higher rate of anorexia. A social worker at the clinic, Julie Dickinson, said she believed the pressures to achieve there were more intense. "The drive for high achievement and excellence and the accompanying competitiveness, which are often part of the ethos of independent schools, feed into perfectionism and encourage the view that high achievement is of prime importance and the only way to be valued as a human being," she said. Bulimia was more evenly spread across public and private schools.

Bulimia nervosa After midnight a silent woman carefully opens the fridge door. She sits alone and stuffs food into herself without pleasure. She gorges on enough for five full meals. She tiptoes to the bathroom, closes the door, and puts her fingers down her throat.

Bulimics are trapped in a cycle of binge eating, guilt, and purging. Figures vary as to how many bulimics there are. Most doctors believe that the problem is much more widespread than anorexia but estimations vary from 3.8 percent to 19 percent in the United States. A 1989 Australian study suggested 1 to 2 percent of the population. A study in Christchurch, New Zealand, revealed only a 0.02 percent rate of bulimia in the general population. Bulimia, some believe, affects 1 in 100 girls. Over three years with proper treatment 80 percent improve, 20 percent persist. Some move to a mixture of anorexia and bulimia. Bulimia is known to be far more common among teenagers and young women, and more likely in women whose weight is deemed relevant to work or to other pursuits such as ballet, acting, and modelling.

Surveys in schools and colleges have turned up results of 4 percent and 10 percent. The problem may be more widespread—bulimia is so secretive it's harder for observers to identify than anorexia.

Bulimics can eat like everybody else but take lots of laxatives to "purge" the food. They can only do so after calories have been absorbed anyway: most bulimics don't know that the weight loss after laxatives and diuretics is not the food but water loss. Bulimics can seem overweight or underweight.

Their condition is characterised by binge eating and then purging the food through vomiting, or laxative and diuretic abuse, exercising, dieting, abuse of diet pills, and fasting. Binge eating is the fast eating of a large amount of food or almost constant nibbling, associated with a sense of being out of control. Food restriction and dieting are also common and so is depression.

Bulimics can display many of the symptoms of anorexia but while anorexics feel in control of their eating and not much else, bulimics feel totally out of control with eating, in contrast to their high-achieving, well-regulated life. They tend to do their bingeing in secret. Some food is chewed and then spat out. A bulimic often diets, and then has to succumb to the body screaming for carbohydrates, and binges. Then the guilt begins and the cycle continues.

The horrible turmoil is a hidden one. Bulimics tend to be passive people who want attention and approval (who doesn't?). Generally speaking, they have some difficulty in being honest about their needs, and they hide their insecurity and self-doubt behind a busy social life.

Apart from misery, physical consequences can include gastrointestinal damage, iron deficiency and poor nutrition, diarrhoea, kidney damage from the diuretic pills, a swollen face, calluses on the hand used to induce vomiting, damage to teeth, mouth, and gullet from stomach acids, fatal stomach rupture, or heart attack. The director of a Sydney eating-disorders clinic says up to half the patients she

Next Thursday at 9.30 A.M. I truly face my problem of 12 years. My fiancé and I are seeking professional therapy at the hospital. Bulimia has, to put it bluntly, shot my self-esteem/self-confidence to shit. And yet people are saying how envious they are of me. I bet they wouldn't be that envious if they knew about the anxiety, frustration, self-hatred, and depression bulimia has scarred me with. I was vomiting six to eight times a day. These eating disorders are so secretive: you deny black and blue there's anything wrong. Soon after the bulimia took hold I added another "tool of removal": laxatives, taking 38 a day (one to two are considered a normal dose). I eventually weaned myself off: being a biologist I know the risks involved. I finally plucked up the courage to tell my fiancé—he found it (and still does) very confusing. Now for the psychological battle that begins next Thursday: wish me luck.

Penny, 27

has seen with bulimia have previously had anorexia.

Dr. Suzanne Abraham of Sydney University, co-author of a book about eating disorders, says that with counselling and nutrition, most patients with eating disorders recover completely. At last, some good news! "But it takes a while to get better," she adds.

Many bulimics can learn how to express their feelings in ways other than those involving food. They learn that they have needs and wants that cannot be met with food, but can be identified and met by other "rewards" in life.

Training for an eating disorder Although common features of women with eating disorders include their unreal expectations of perfection and difficulty in accepting natural weight gains in the teenage years, that doesn't mean that all ambitious high achievers are anorexics or bulimics. But every authority on eating disorders says parents and teachers should not pressure students to unrealistic goals or to perfection.

What, then, to make of the special program started at a Sydney elementary school where girls, between 6 and 12 years old, have been chosen to attend a special gymnastics school to prepare them for the Olympics in the year 2000? According to a newspaper report, the girls will be "kept together with their teacher...while they are groomed to be great athletes." Leanne Schmidt, the girls' teacher and a former gymnast, said she did not go through puberty until she was 18 and a half, when she stopped training and grew almost 12 inches in three months.

Here are little girls who will be taught that becoming a woman, getting periods and the change in body shape, is their enemy; that to be unnaturally stunted is good; and that the definition of their success will be measured by whether they become Olympians.

Even if the girls do not develop eating disorders, how will this delaying of puberty affect them? Can you imagine the outcry if a Sydney school announced that it was gathering a team of 12 young boys, aged 6 to 12, and delaying the boys' natural development until they were 18 to keep their voices high so they could sing soprano and be the right height as a special choir to sing at the opening of the 2000 Olympics?

The Australian Institute of Sport's own psychologist, Jeff Bond, said in 1992 that he believed dozens of Australia's top athletes were suffering from anorexia and bulimia. "I'm talking about the national and international level," he specified.

Mr. Bond said, "There is a much, much stronger emphasis almost year by year now on power-to-weight ratios and low body fat and so on." He told the *Sydney Morning Herald* that anorexia tended to be a feature of distance and artistic sports such as gymnastics, but bulimia was more prevalent across the board.

I asked Mr. Bond about the school for gymnasts, the delaying of puberty for gymnasts, and whether this was acceptable policy. He said, "It's inevitable, I'm not sure it's acceptable. As a parent, as a humanist, I'd say it's not acceptable. As a realist, working within the system of elite sport, we [the sports psychologists] try to cushion it as best we can."

Mr. Bond said the stopping of periods through stress from training, as well as lowered body fat, was "an accepted thing in elite sport."

Mr. Bond also said that, as a psychologist within the system, he worked to try and make athletes aware that they were just going through a phase in their lives, making great sacrifices, and that they would move on to another phase. He said sometimes the athletes were not aware of all the sacrifices they were making. (I would say that is particularly true for a 6-year-old girl enrolled in a gymnasts' school.)

When you watch the Olympics in the year 2000, think of what those little girls have been put through, paid for with their government's money.

Ballet According to a professor of psychiatry at Sydney University, there is evidence that ballet dancers are particularly prone to developing anorexia and bulimia nervosa. He says, "Their ballet teachers ask them to keep weight levels which are physiologically abnormal. There's a lot of unhappiness amongst many health professionals about the poor advice that many ballet teachers give their students." Sydney ballet teacher Virginia Gallagher says she guards against the problem with her students because of her own experience as a ballet student. She was given amphetamines and developed bulimia like three others in her class; another two had anorexia.

There is a long tradition of these destructive requirements. Gelsey Kirkland, one of ballet guru George Balanchine's students, recalls in her autobiography, *Dancing on My Grave*, a moment when Balanchine halted a class to inspect her. "With his knuckles, he thumped on my sternum and down my rib cage, clucking his tongue and remarking 'Must see the bones.' I was less than 100 pounds even then," she wrote. "He did not merely say 'Eat less.' He said 'Eat nothing!'"

The acclaimed Mark Morris Dance Company has rejected the narrow ideal and shows the way

My bulimia has worsened over the past year and I have been in the hospital once. Most of the time I feel like a big fat loser because I don't know many winners who stand over the washbasin four or five times a day with their hand down their throat. I know taking Ipecac weakens your heart and diet pills dull your brain but if they worked I'd still be taking them. My circulation is stuffed, my face and throat are always puffy, my skin always blotchy, and I have broken capillaries from having my head down too often, not to mention scars on my right hand's first two knuckles. Sorry about the pleasant description but the point I'm trying to get across (even to myself) is that bulimia is a dead end. I look even further from the models I was trying to emulate at the start.

Pamela, 17

of the future. It has dancers of all different shapes and sizes. "[Critics] have always said we have big butts," Mark Morris agrees. "We have big butts. The point is: who CARES."

Modelling Penelope Tree, one of the original "waif" models from the 1960s, now says she was anorexic as a famous model. She started dieting at boarding school because she felt emotionally abandoned. She was 36 before she got bulimia under control. She identifies "the sad and pitiful irony of beautiful models in beautiful expensive magazines who are destroying themselves for other people."

She remains convinced that having an eating disorder is rewarded by society. It is seen as glamorous, enviable, professionally successful, and financially rewarding for models and actors. She believes that women are trapped into being thinner for other women as part of the competition and that the industry which encourages the unreal thinness is bigger than all of us. "But steps can be taken on an individual basis," she says. "Young women, especially adolescents, have to be taught how to feel good about themselves. You have to find something worthwhile to fill the hole of emptiness and confusion that confronts us all when we are growing up."

Role models Several observers say that a major contributing factor to eating disorders is the widening gap between reality and the cultural ideal. A Melbourne psychiatrist wrote to an Australian newspaper saying he could not "remain silent while ever-increasing numbers" of young women are referred to him for therapy for their eating disorders. "Surely it is time for those responsible for influencing our young women and for setting the so-called 'ideal' to demonstrate some responsibility and encourage the use of more normal representatives of the female community to sell fashion... It is with great alarm that I have noticed the fashion industry's recent move towards promoting the image of the undernourished, 'waif-like gamine' as the latest pinnacle of perfection for women." He linked these cultural pressures to the women with eating disorders.

Schoolgirls Jacqueline McArthur and Caitlin MacLeod also wrote to the newspaper, saying, "Lining our walls are *Elle* cutouts of often adolescent *boys* stylised and photographed in women's clothing to shape the unattainable ideal in our minds. The toilets no longer smell of smoke, but of vomit. Last year a girl was hospitalised with anorexia nervosa, only to appear six months later gracing the pages of *Dolly* magazine."

The editor of British *Vogue*, Alexandra Shulman, defended her use of waif models by saying, "I don't understand the fuss. It has been proved over and over again that anorexia and bulimia have nothing to do with fashion pictures. Models have always been thin. Kate Moss is shorter than most models, but no thinner." That last sentence is laughable to anyone who has seen pictures of Kate Moss. But perhaps it is too easy for Ms. Shulman to say that fashion pictures do not cause anorexia and bulimia. They are, at least according to the evidence of many young women struggling with eating disorders and their doctors and therapists, part of their problem.

Several eating-disorders clinics will not allow any women's magazines on the premises. And the National Association of Anorexia Nervosa and Associated Disorders has successfully lobbied against the use of dangerous advertising slogans like "You can never be too rich or too thin."

Families and friends An eating-disorders clinic suggests the following for friends and parents to help prevent anorexia and bulimia:

- Share the information you have about the dangers of dieting.
- Help others to understand the purposes of advertising images, and why they must not be taken to heart.
- Do not push children or friends to excel in sports and other areas.
- Examine your own motives for wanting those associated with you to excel.
- Adolescents need a mix of rules and freedoms in their lives, without being overprotected or abandoned to fend for themselves. Let friends and children work through their pain and problems by themselves, with your support. Your role is to love, support, and encourage. Help young people to understand the difference between a good diet (nutrition) and dieting. Avoid encouraging young people to lose weight.
- Be a good role model for other women. Avoid criticising your own body. Stop talking about physical appearance and diets. Express admiration for healthy bodies, even if they are not thin.
- Be a good role model for other men. Avoid criticising women who do not meet your standards of physical beauty. Don't encourage your wife, girlfriend, sister, or daughter to lose weight because you think it would make *you* feel better. ▶

> • Talk to friends and children about why they want to lose weight. If it is because of feelings of inadequacy, deal with those issues. If the feelings continue, find a counsellor who is trained to work with eating disorders. The anorexia and bulimia nervosa groups have more information for family and friends.

Getting help Because the psychological reasons for eating disorders can be so ingrained, many people who have had anorexia and bulimia have relapses and need further help throughout their lives. Others may want to head off the problem before it gets overwhelming.

> Laxatives make ya bum sting.
>
> Georgina, 15

A range of treatments is available for each disorder, including group therapy, psychotherapy and counselling, nutritional counselling, assertion training, family therapy, and hospitalisation only in very severe cases.

People may take time to find the right therapist. One ex-bulimic encourages those who need help not to be discouraged if the first doctor or psychiatrist doesn't understand the problem or is contemptuous of it. It is very important that you contact an anorexia and bulimia support group so you can talk to people who really understand and will not judge you.

Many people have been cured of their eating disorders; others

I am 24 years old and have been bulimic for approximately six to seven years. I was anorexic at 106 pounds. I was running the family home at 11 and sexually abused by my uncle at three years old and I was always a fat child. I remembered when I was twenty-one. My mother and sister were both models: I was acknowledged for being clever but ugly. Nearly every girl I know has or has had an eating disorder: three bulimic, one anorexic, three bulimic and anorexic, one obese, and four normal. It appears the younger girls are the more prone to disorders. My older friends have grown up with less pressure or have just learned to accept their bodies the way they are.

Rula

Bulimia is a struggle every day. In the end it gets me nowhere: I have achieved no significant weight loss from this. This eating disorder is caused mostly by my desire to be thinner but after thinking it over I've discovered that in a small way it is also attributed to my need for more attention because I live in a large family where there isn't a lot of attention to go around.

Haylie, 19

problem as serious. Therapists can have their own problems and biases.

Dr. Clark from the Sydney clinic says the best place to start is your local doctor. Ask for a full examination and, if necessary, referral to an eating-disorders clinic. "If you feel too heavy or too light, seek help or information," he says. Most women are treated as private patients or as hospital outpatients.

Your local doctor may not be experienced in treating eating disorders but can refer you for help or get instructions on how to help you. Nutritionists at eating-disorders clinics, women's health centres, and the National Center for Nutrition can also help you. Women's health centres will be able to refer you to a body-image group or eating-disorders group.

have their eating disorders as the background to their lives, but manageable. Many are particularly helped by making the decision to go to therapy—not as a failure, but as a positive step towards helping themselves and becoming well, a new challenge.

Don't go to a therapist who offers you a quick cure, or a better cure for more money, or who talks only of willpower or does not see the

When asking bulimics to define bulimia, the replies were all associated with feelings, or the effects bulimia had on their lives. Vomiting and laxative abuse were not mentioned... [Comments include:]

—It's not living, just existing.

—If you are not doing it, you are thinking about doing it.

—It stops you from living and appreciating the moment. It is paralysing fear.

—Chaotic, not living.

—It blocks out life, it's not living.

—My personal definition of bulimia is when a person's relation to food becomes the medium used in which to express repressed thoughts and feelings.

Lui Suit, bulimia research project,
Murdoch University, Perth

Anorexia and bulimia groups can send you information, give advice over the phone, and refer you for further help. You may be surprised to find so many people who share your experiences.

Several private psychiatrists are working in the field of eating disorders. Some of them have personal theories about the causes of anorexia or bulimia which they explore during sessions. While some of these therapists may be very helpful for some women, they are generally not able to help with nutritional advice and programs.

As the causes of the disorders are multi-dimensional, so may be the treatments.

People with eating disorders can feel alone in the wilderness. Actually the wilderness is pretty crowded these days. You can learn to read the signs—especially the ones which say "Wrong way: go back!"

Contacts

These are just a few of the support groups throughout the United States and Canada which will send you information or help you on the phone. They can also refer you to clinics, individual practitioners, and hospital programs near you:

American Anorexia/Bulimia Association, Inc.
293 Central Park West
Suite 1R
New York, NY 10024
Phone: (212)501-8351

Anorexia/Bulimia Treatment and Education Center
621 South New Ballas Road
Suite 7019B
St. Louis, MO 63141
Phone: (800)222-2832

Help Anorexia
5143 Overland Avenue
Culver City, CA 90230
Phone: (213)837-5445 or (213)836-1191 ▶

Anorexia Nervosa and Related Eating Disorders
Box 5102
Eugene, OR 97405
Phone: (503)344-1144

National Anorexia Aid Society
Box 29461
Columbus, OH 43229
Phone: (614)816-6810
National Association of Anorexia and Associated Disorders
Box 7
Highland Park, IL 60035
Phone: (708)831-3438

National Eating Disorders Organization
Harding Hospital
445 E. Granville Road
Worthington, OH 43085
Phone: (614)436-1112

Health departments

Ask for the nearest clinic or hospital with an eating-disorders
unit or services. Unless your life is in immediate danger you can
almost certainly visit the hospital for treatment without having to
stay overnight.

Further reading

Marlene Boskind-White and William C. White, Jr., *Bulimarexia*
(New York: W.W. Norton, 1991).

Dr. Phyllis Butow, Jillian Ball, and Fiona Place, *When Eating is
Everything: How to Overcome Your Eating Problems and Change
Your Life* (New York: Doubleday, 1991).

Dr. Judith Rodin, *Body Traps: How to Overcome Your Body* ▶

Obsessions and Liberate the Real You (New York: William Morrow, 1992).

Matra Robertson, *Starving in the Silences: An Explanation of Anorexia Nervosa* (Sydney: Allen & Unwin, 1992). Very academic.

M. Siegal, J. Brisman, and M. Weinshal, *Surviving an Eating Disorder: Strategies for Families and Friends* (New York: Harper & Row, 1988).
J. Hirschmann and L. Zaphiropoulos, *Are You Hungry?* (New York: Random House, 1985).

Hara Estroff Morano, *Style Is Not a Size: Looking and Feeling Great in the Body You Have* (New York: Bantam, 1991).

L. Newman, *Some Body to Love* (Chicago: Third Side Press, 1991).

Geneen Roth, *Compulsory Eating* (New York: Macmillan, 1982).

Geneen Roth, *Breaking Free from Compulsive Eating* (New York: Macmillan, 1984).

Ira M. Sacker, M.D. and Marc A. Zimmer, Ph.D., *Dying to Be Thin: Understanding and Defeating Anorexia Nervosa and Bulimia: A Practical Lifesaving Guide* (New York: Warner Books, 1987).

Kim Chernin, *The Hungry Self: Women, Eating and Identity* (New York: Times Books, 1985).

Caroline Miller, *My Name Is Caroline* (New York: Doubleday, 1988).

Katherine Gilday, *The Famine Within* (1990, a 90-minute video available from Direct Cinema, P.O. Box 10003, Santa Monica, CA 90410).

Exercise

Too little Recent research by the U.S. Centers for Disease Control and Prevention showed that only 25 percent of female high-school seniors exercise regularly, compared with 50 percent of boys the same age. The researchers believe that girls are becoming less active and do less exercise as they get older. Only 36 percent of elementary- and secondary-school students have daily phys ed classes.

A fifth of all adults spend leisure time in a physical activity, a fourth are completely inactive, and the rest are considered "inadequately active" by the Centers for Disease Control. The statistics show that 75 percent of people who begin an exercise program give up within a year. We're a proud nation of lazy, TV-watching slugs.

The Australian National Heart Foundation's "Active Girls Can Do Anything" campaign (although I would advise active girls not to pee standing up if they can avoid it) was launched in 1993 because nearly half of Australia's women die of heart and blood vessel disease, and they reckon a lot of this is preventable. Not death itself, though; so far as we know, this is not yet preventable.

Anyway, according to their figures there are more unfit girls than boys, and too many girls are being discouraged from sports. They get less recognition and support than boys for their achievement and effort. Which is a complete rip-off, because girls who don't play sports are often less healthy, less confident, and don't like them-selves as much as girls who do.

We are up against it here, when less than 5 percent of newspapers' sports pages are devoted to women's sports. In the last Olympics there were 159 men's events and 86 women's events. The National Federation of State High School Associations reported an all-time high of 2.1 million girls involved in high- school athletics in 1993–94. Even so, girls remain much less active than boys: 3.5 million boys took part in high-school athletics in the same year. Girls were mainly involved with basketball, track and field, volleyball, and fast-pitch softball, with soccer, tennis, swimming, and diving next in popularity.

Women's and girls' participation has increased enormously since a federal law was introduced in 1972 guaranteeing equal rights and funding for women's sports. In 1971 only 294,000 high- school girls played any sport.

But it is still harder to interest girls than boys in getting sweaty. A 1990 survey of 11,000 students by the Centers for Disease Control found that 35 percent of ninth-grade girls had 20 minutes of "vigorous activity" three times a week, compared with 53 percent of their male classmates. The numbers decreased to 25 and 50 percent when the students reached their senior yorear.

Inactivity gets worse as women get older. "Women aged 20 to 50 are very busy with their families and careers and they don't take optimal care of themselves," said Dr. Walter C. Willett at Harvard University's School of Public Health. "They're not carving out that 20 minutes a day for exercise."

On average, girls tend to be less effective than boys in some sporting skills, such as throwing balls. There is no physical explanation for this. It is about girls not being encouraged and taught the same way. And the aerobic fitness (heart-lung working capacity) of girls starts declining, on average, after the age of 12. Which, *not* coinci-

> I think that in *Dolly* mag they should have a complete lift-out on what exercises to do for the different parts of the body where people want to lose weight...hips, legs, stomach. I dislike my hips, butt, and thighs, they all need a good workout. I look in all the mags and I wish I looked like the models but life goes on!
>
> "Keen," 13

dentally, is the same age that self-esteem generally starts to plummet through the floor.

According to the Australian National Heart Foundation, girls are more likely to underrate their performance than boys. If a girl and a boy throw a ball exactly the same distance, the boy is more likely to say, "That was great," and the girl will think, "Not good enough, I shall go and attempt to drown myself in the science laboratory." Once they stop, girls seem to get shyer about starting again, being seen by others to make mistakes, and their bodies being seen by others, particularly their new, unfamiliar bodies with breasts and hips. (This is not helped by the taunts of other girls and boys, who are made frenzied and nasty by their own puberty freakouts.)

Girls tend to see sport as a participation, affiliation with others, and a team activity; boys tend to see it more as achievement based, a view more richly rewarded in the past.

We have to be more like the boys if we're going to get in there and enjoy ourselves. Girls tend not to participate if their skill level is low, whereas boys are braver, more likely to have a go and learn from their mistakes. We have to demand the space we need, as space and equipment for girls to play sports are often much less than those allocated for boys—in schools which are not allowed to do this but do it anyway. This doesn't mean we have to necessarily play sports *with* the boys, which can be a torrid and bruising affair, but we should get the same equipment to, ahem, if you'll excuse the expression, play with ourselves.

We can learn from boys and men how to get up and keep going when we've scraped a knee and missed a goal (without taking on angry feelings at ourselves). We can learn from boys and men how to go on when we're not immediately good at something. Actually we can learn from some men's leagues how to go on when we're never really good at something. We can do it for the fun of it, even if we'll never hit the top of the ladder.

And maybe some could learn from us that exercising doesn't always have to be only about winning. There's belly dancing, basketball strategy meetings, archery, and long walks looking at the world and taking time out to smell the roses, as long as we don't get thorns up our nostrils.

Too much Too much exercise can encourage some people to become anorexic. A professor from the Department of Psychiatry at Sydney University says that once a person's weight falls below a certain level, behaviour patterns become obvious—the over-exerciser stops eating, the overdieter starts exercising.

For the last two years I've been doing 100 sit-ups, give or take 50, at least five nights a week, but my weight hasn't changed once. I can't stand it. I've come to realise it's mainly got to do with genetics. My parents are heavily built but still healthy.

Mardi, 17

The professor noted that the overexercisers began their regime because they were concerned about their weight and shape, whereas many anorexics stopped eating properly because of anxiety and other problems.

One kind of overactivity, he said, "followed too literally the advice of magazines that suggested 'never sit if you can stand, never stand if you can walk, never walk if you can run.'" Sufferers of this disorder sometimes get into a complicated, endless "debt" system, where they eat to reward themselves for exercising, but exercise to punish the eating. This can lead to overexercising anorexia patients being finally admitted to a hospital or other treatment centre in a far worse state than those who were not exercising as well as starving.

(One of the things about exercising is that if you wear polyester hot-pink tights for hours on a stationary bicycle you will probably get raging thrush over half of your body, but yet another thing is that if you exercise, you will also have to eat extra protein, iron, calcium, and carbohydrates and drink a lot of water.)

Some women look at those charts which tell you how much energy you have to expend to "lose" some food you've eaten. This is often expressed thus: "One carrot. Must run around the house for four days and then cycle interstate." Forget these stupid, STUPID charts, which completely ignore the fact that we need the food to make our bodies like, you know, work? Every piece of food you eat is used by the body to make the skin system work, help pump the blood around and replace cells and walk and talk and grow hair. Food has work to do. The equation of eat it and be punished or eat it and then work it off is just crazy. If you see one of these charts, do not approach it; it may be charming and dangerous. Cut it out and feed it to the dog.

Former middle-distance runner Michelle Baumgartner recalls that her strict dieting and athletic training stopped her menstruating at 19. At her peak of athletic success her body fat was an astonishing 8 percent; women should be 22 to 30 percent. "It took me five years from the time I stopped training to recover," she said. "I suffered from all sorts of problems but my coach and people around would tell me that I looked great and to keep pushing myself...I was underweight and sick and nobody seemed to notice. But if I didn't win it was my fault...[We used to joke] how fantastic it was we didn't have to go through periods. I now realise I was lucky to retire when I did." Another former running mate had four bone grafts before she was 26 to try and correct the problems.

Overexercise can thin the bones, just as anorexia does, making the body vulnerable to osteoporosis. Some young female athletes are left with the chalky, brittle bones of women in their 70s or 80s. Under intense pressures, female athletes lose a lot of weight, developing eating disorders, stress fractures, menstrual disorders, and osteoporosis.

High-impact aerobics and other exercise on a hard surface can cause jarring of joints, tearing of tissue, and damage to the inner ear.

Another big drawback of exercise is that it has spawned a repulsive and often risky mountain of celebrity exercise videos by every white-grinned thin movie star, rock star, and model with advice from often dubious "personal trainers" (torturers) focusing on bits of the body—stomach, bottom, hips, thighs. These videos can damage your body, and following their regimes can have very little to do with real fitness.

Anyway, isn't it a bit lonely, just you and a video?

This is related to the Scary Gyms Full of Scary People Syndrome—intimidating men with unnaturally wide necks who smell like chemicals when they sweat (that'll be your steroids) and underfed women who look at you strangely if you have legs bigger than breadsticks, especially if you're wearing shorts and a T-shirt which says "Pre-Menstrual As Anything." Some gyms cater to people who are not muscle-bound or vampirical.

The obsession with exercise has spawned some very stupid

marketing ideas: *Allure* magazine says we should wear waterproof makeup while sweating (bad idea). A model used to illustrate the magazine's special on exercise looks to be either extraordinarily naturally thin and bony or else the victim of an eating or exercising disorder: you can see the outline of her bones underneath her skin. The caption reads, "Fat chance. Sure, low-intensity is just as good as high-intensity exercise—but you have to do it longer." There is a makeup credit but we cannot see the model's face.

You know those exercises you see in magazines with a maniacally grinning instructor demonstrating each one, or a drawing of a woman who in real life would be 9 feet tall and weigh as much as a pocket packet of tissues? You're better off going to an aerobics class with a qualified, sensible teacher or a low-key yoga instructor to show you exactly the right way to do them. Otherwise you may wrench something, or topple over, or just generally make a dork of yourself doing six months of exercises that don't actually exercise anything except your time. Or you could hurt yourself if you develop a bad habit in your own lounge room, such as bouncing on a stretching movement or watching sitcoms with "family values."

Many of these exercises in magazines concentrate on one area of your body, usually thighs, bottom, and stomach, but sometimes other bits (arms, even). This kind of obsession with one area of the body encourages you to think weirdly about yourself. People will greet you, "Hi, Jane," and you will say, "Say hello to my biceps, too, they get lonely." And doing those sorts of exercises takes time and leaves the other bits to get mouldy and neglected.

Enough It is generally accepted that we would all feel better about ourselves and be healthier if we exercised three times a week. Each time, the exercise should have us breathing much faster than normal for at least 20 minutes, and 40 minutes if possible. Beginners should work up to these levels over time.

Why exercise? Exercise reduces stress and tiredness. Also, you can stop when it hurts, which is more than you can say for life in general. Also, you can choose the best kind for you. This means that if walking up and down three stairs at the gym is boring you until you want to shriek, shriek, *shriek*, you can go and learn the Lambada next door.

It means that if you can't get the motivation to go and inter- act with a machine three times a week, you can join a team and play sport with humanoids. Ex- ercise makes you more aware of your own body and makes you think of yourself more as a whole being than a collection of parts, or a brain followed around by all that baggage underneath.

The American Heart Associa- tion, which is always banging on about getting more exercise, lists several benefits including improved concentration, relaxation, less tension, sleeping better, improved posture, strength, fitness, im- proved digestion and easier breathing, greater confidence, feeling happy and relaxed, a healthier blood cholesterol level, lower blood pressure, stronger bones, longer life, and less likelihood of a heart attack. Well, that's a bonus.

There are less obvious benefits, such as developing friendships and work contacts through sports, opportunities to learn how to deal with success and failure and a whole lot of other gobbledegook about personal challenges and team efforts and stuff that kind of makes me sick so I won't bore you with it.

Getting started It is ex- tremely hard to get motivated, un-

Australian champion swimmer Lisa Curry exercises for five hours a day. We interviewed Jamie Lee Curtis who was meant to have the "perfect body." She worked out four hours a day for that body. Now she has a child and better things to do with herself.

Diane Parks, Australian editor, *Slimming* magazine

less you're like Madonna and have a personal trainer, which is just like hiring somebody to shout at you "Get up, you lazy grizzly bear!" and then run around after thinking up other insults and saying, "Hup two three four," until you strangle them with something made of Lycra and get off on justifiable homicide and *still* have to pay them $100 an hour. Anyway, other than that, you may, like somebody I know not entirely unadjacent to *me*, rather lie in bed and see how the dream ends. Or lie in bed and not see how the dream ends. But, basically, for whatever reason seems closest to hand at the time, lie in bed.

Some ways to get around this motivational problem include paying gym membership in advance (this rarely works, you just lose your money and feel cross with yourself for not going); making a time to walk, run, or swim with friends; and playing a team sport so you are in a group that relies on each other to turn up for training and matches.

Another problem with exercise is that if you've never done any, and you suddenly start doing a great deal of it, your body can become totally affronted, and you might die. The way to avoid this is to lead your body into the subject very gently so it hardly gets huffy at all, and before it knows it, it's having its fingertips introduced to the toes and the blood is pumping around, heartily making itself acquainted with all the extremities.

Another drawback of suddenly beginning to exercise can be injury. This can be avoided by kitting yourself out correctly, with the right shoesies and things and, if circumstances require, helmets, kneepads, mouthguards, private health insurance, and an ambulance at the bottom of the hill.

You can also avoid injury by not playing the more brutal sports in which skill is less important than the level of truly innovative violence and opportunities for spinal injury and blindness. These include one of the codes of rugby, I can't remember which one, but it's probably the one in which they gaffer-tape their ears to their heads in case they get ripped off, and also low-grade ice hockey, and any game in which the opposition has expressed an interest in examining your entrails.

There is quite a lot of sexism in sport, which discourages women from participating and pushes them into early spectatorhood. Part of this is an uneven distribution of funds to sport by schools, governments, and sponsors. Another is that girls have been less encouraged to do daring things. In the past, boys were supposed to do strong, exhibitionist, dangerous things (weightlifting, football), and girls were supposed to do flouncy, pretty things (gymnastics, ballet). This is changing, and champion girl and women surfers, in-line skaters, softball players, martial artists, runners, jumpers, basketballers, soccer players, and their sisters in all codes are waiting for you to join them. Just make sure you're fit enough to run if any of them asks to see your entrails.

But we can fight the discrimination and discouragement, and get out there and get the benefits. (Some trumpet music here, please.) Even though women form a smaller part of the Australian Olympic team than men, they have always won more medals proportionately. And we don't even have to be Olympians. We don't even have to want to. I certainly don't—those opening-ceremony uniforms

are usually embarrassing. (Whoops, sorry, I just channelled the fashion police.)

If you are discriminated against because you cannot use the facilities of a sporting club, or you're forced to be an associate member, or you're not being given access to equipment at school, you can lodge a complaint, or ring for advice from the Civil Rights Commission or Department of Education's Office of Civil Rights. You may not choose the right exercise genre first time. In fact, it would be amazing if you did not have to try out a few things to see what you liked best. The second time I tried aerobics it was an Afro-Brazilian class where the teacher, Mistress Maria, set a literally blistering pace which involved exhorting the class to do things like: "Now, in time to the music, place your left ankle over your right shoulder and leave it in the far corner of the gymnasium. Now do 800 push-ups. Maybe 900. I don't know yet."

(A word of warning. Golf. Golf is exercise and golf is stupid. Do not let this put you off exercise itself.)

Types of exercise
Aerobic exercise Lifts your heart rate, and makes you sweat and breathe quicker. This means stuff like jogging, walking quickly, riding a bike, skipping, aerobics, aquarobics, running around a sports field without stopping, and fleeing from a house where they are playing Barry Manilow songs.

Isometric exercise Weight training, often on machines, using small groups of muscles at a time.

Just stuff Walking home from the bus, answering the telephone, ironing, shopping, hanging out the washing, lifting kids, chasing kids, cooking, gardening, using the stairs, living. This actually takes up most of our body fuel: it is the bulk of our energy expenditure.

Vigorous relaxing A more Eastern approach emphasising balance, economy of motion, centring, and harmonious use of the body—for example, yoga, tai-chi, martial arts.

Energetic exercise Abandoned sex and wild dancing.

Guru exercise This is when you slavishly follow the directions of one instructor or discipline. Don't forget you can keep an open mind and choose the best bits from anywhere you like. This is called Buffet Exercise. No it's not, I just made that up. Maybe I should have a video.

Simple calorie burning This determined, compulsive exercise is aimed only at losing weight, instead of using all parts of the body and warming up and cooling down. Often people who do this look kind of frenzied and desperate.

Fun Things you do with friends, or relatives, or the dog. Frisbee, chatting while walking with a friend, splashing around with an old canoe, learning country-and-western dancing; anything involving a "hit and giggle."

Pretendy exercise This is where they strap you to a table and it moves your body for you. Or using those little electrode pads which are taped to your thighs and stomach which are supposed to shape, sculpt, or tone your body, according to the brochures. What they do is send little electric impulses into your body. There is usually also a lot of guff about microsecond pulses, monophasic wave forms, and longitudinal padding of the muscle. It's a gimmick that claims to "condition" your body's muscles by jiggling them about with electronic impulses. Often billed as some sort of workout on a couch, it is no substitute for exercise and does nothing for heart-lung fitness.

Avoid exercising which divorces you from yourself (bear with me, I'm not going all New Age hippie on you). Choose an exercise thingy (I hesitate to use the word *plan*; I have always hesitated to use a word like *plan*, and I'm sorry but I just can't start now)...choose an exercise thingy that's fun, that's about *you* exercising. Not one that's about: "My right thigh is now exercising; now my left thigh. Now my butt is exercising. At about half-past three, my left bicep will be distinguishing itself." Also, do *not* weigh yourself and freak out. Muscle weighs more than fat. It doesn't mean you're overweight. Anyway, you know what you should do with bathroom scales. Sledgehammers ahoy!

Beware of exercise and jargon that encourage body hatred, or that see the body as the enemy. So avoid "bottom burners," "stomach crunchers," and such careless nasty talk about yourself.

The very best magical thing about exercising I will admit that exercise does have one perfectly magical effect. It makes you feel better about yourself. It makes you feel good about yourself. Exercise, if I could just make things utterly clear, raises your self-esteem. Just about any form of exercise will do this except one where you're surrounded with neurotic people in mauve leotards who are comparing people's body shapes and making you feel inadequate so they can feel better about themselves, or except when the main reason for exercise is that your body is seen as the enemy: "I have to get rid of these hips."

And this feeling better about yourself happens *regardless* of your weight or shape. If you're a size 16 and you exercise regularly and you are meant to be a size 16 and you stay a size 16, you will *like yourself more*.

This is the one truly fabulous thing about exercise, and it is just a great shame that it is not really something you can do while you are asleep.

Further information

The American Heart Association has enough information on all this stuff to choke a Clydesdale, and they have free pamphlets to send to individuals and schools and videos to lend to schools. They have branches all over the country.

Your local Department of Parks and Recreation office will have a list of activities and classes such as yoga, dance, swimming, and aerobics. Ask about the qualifications of your instructor. Most of these classes are inexpensive

The Parks and Recreation people will also have information about sporting groups in the area. You can join by yourself, or with a friend.

Check out local hiking clubs. Many of them put together groups for organised walking or other activities.

Each state and city government department which looks after sport can give you information on funding and other opportunities for women.

See the lists at the end of the book.

chapter three

What is normal?

Do I have normal breasts?

32B or not 32B Unless you have breasts shaped like question marks, they're probably normal. Most women have a right breast larger than their left. Just about everyone will develop stretch marks with their first breast growth spurt. Later, hairs will grow around the nipple. Normal breasts can be very small or very large (girls and women with larger breasts can have neck, chest, and back pain from bra straps holding the weight and suffer cruel comments and rude stares).

These women at the outer edge of the normal range can find it difficult to get bras to fit them—not because they're not "normal" but because the manufacturers don't make the same profits from the women who ask for a bra size they don't sell the most of: 32B or not 32B, that is their question.

Breasts are for feeling good when they're touched and for breastfeeding, whatever their size. Small breasts may be easier for breastfeeding because there is less to get in the way when a baby is suckling. Breastfeeding provides natural immunities against sickness

My breasts often seem too small.

Fran, 19

I'm as flat as a pancake. All the other girls my age have breasts and I don't. It's very embarrassing. PS: How do you get into this modelling business?

Judy, 13

for a baby, as well as being its only food in the early months. After breastfeeding the breasts may be smaller and less outwardly pointing than before. With age, especially after menopause, the breasts become less plumped out.

Breasts can be round, hard, soft, lumpy, irregularly shaped, shaped like test tubes, large, small, shaped like quinces, shaped like ferret noses, pointed in opposite directions, high, low, bounce from side to side or up and down, with cleavage, far apart, with freckles, with pink nipples and areolae (the coloured area around the protruding nipple), browner nipples and areolae (especially after pregnancy), wide oval areolae, small circular areolae. The areolae have little bumps on them. Some people develop a third or extra nipples underneath the breasts or on the stomach, which are often mistaken for moles. Some can tie their breasts in a knot behind their head. This is not recommended on public transport.

I think the comedian Denis Leary speaks for most men when he says, "I don't understand the fascination with breast implants. I like the real thing, no matter what the size. I like big ones. I like small ones. I think I even like the smaller ones better than the big ones. I love all shapes, all sizes. I love the ones that are shaped like golf balls, I love the ones that are shaped like teardrops. I like the melons and the pears, the footballs and the ferns. I love the ones shaped like LBJ's head. I love them all, as long as they 're real." Thank you, Denis.

◎

Lumps and bumps You should get to know the shape and feel of your breasts, which may be naturally slightly lumpy. Then, when you examine your breasts by look and touch after each period (when they are least likely to be retaining fluid) you can notice any changes. You can develop breast cancer at any age. But it's rarer in women under 30, and more common in women as they get older and in those who have a history of it in the family.

A breast lump may be an early sign of a problem that can be cured easily or it may be nothing to worry about. But if it does develop—and size is no indication of how dangerous a lump is—it could result in incurable cancer. The American Cancer Society slogan is: "Early detection is the best protection."

About 180,000 women were diagnosed with breast cancer in the United States in 1994. Many will eventually die of it but live normal lives for another 20 or 30 years. Others will be "cured," if they have come early for treatment. Thousands of women don't know they have it. More than 45,000 American women die of breast cancer each year. Others with advanced cancer can be cured but the radiation therapy can make them unable to have children afterwards.

Many women have the small lump removed rather than an entire breast. Tell all the women in your family, especially those who are over 40, that they should get an examination at a Planned Parenthood clinic or from their gynaecologist. A breast examination can be done once a year by your doctor at the same time as a Pap smear, or during a visit for something else.

So if a lump appears, go and have it looked at. You won't need surgery to confirm a diagnosis. The doctor will put a fine needle into the lump and take out some fluid. It can be a pretty scary thing to go through, so take a friend or relative in with you if you like.

You might have heard that Asian women are at less risk. This is only true for women of Asian origin in their country of heritage and eating a traditional diet.

There is an opinion that breastfeeding and the caressing, manipulating, and stimulation of breasts and nipple help to guard against cancer. (Hmmm. Alright!) It is known that pregnancy does something to breasts to make them less likely to develop cancer, unless there is a history of it in the family. And yet the U.S. Centers for Disease Control found that three-quarters of cases were in women with no publicised risk factors. The only real way to stop it is eternal vigilance and to get any lumps checked out immediately—weeks can be crucial.

Doctors are still not certain whether the family history of shared breast cancer is due to heredity or shared environment or diet. A breast cancer gene was recently identified. But it's estimated that an inherited gene causes 10 percent at most of the breast cancer cases diagnosed each year. The latest tip is that a high-fibre diet may help. The jump in breast cancer in the last 20 years is often attributed partly to a higher-fat diet. Also many researchers in the United States now believe that the higher breast cancer rate (and higher rates of other cancers) may be due to the levels of agricultural pesticide residues in meat and other foods. There is increasing evidence that carcinogens come from various sources such as industry, its production and toxic waste, and pesticides.

These researchers suggest—and it can't hurt—that we should get rid of all the synthetic chemicals possible in our immediate and community environments, especially organochlorins such as DDT, PCBs, CFCs, and dioxins. (According to the Environmental Protection Agency, counties with hazardous waste sites are 6.5 times more likely to have high breast cancer rates than other counties. Two counties routinely saturated with aerial spraying of the pesticide DDT during the 1950s report the highest breast cancer rates.)

Despite the money spent on breast cancer, most is going on the idea of "cures" and detection of a problem already there; the emphasis has not been on prevention. One of the best steps towards preventing cancers may be to join an environmental group that works against the dangerous use and dumping of toxic chemicals, and find a book of hints for "greener" living.

cross your heart BRA

Inverted nipples One in ten women has inverted nipples. This means the nipple is in recess rather than protruding. Most women find theirs can be popped out for breastfeeding. A small safe plastic cup with a vacuum effect can be used to draw out the nipple and "train" it to point outwards. This can also be done by gently pulling the nipple out each day. ("*Hello* there!") Some doctors may suggest a surgical alternative but that should be a very last resort. If your nipple suddenly inverts, having never done so before, see a doctor.

◎

Bust firming "I must, I must improve my bust," goes the desperate chant of women doing silly pectoral exercises that cannot "improve" or enlarge breasts. This desperation can lead them to frighteningly expensive and totally useless creams like the thrilling Guaranteed Sabrina Cream and the New Curvy Girl Method which were flogged in *True Confessions* magazines and comics of the 1950s and 1960s.

"You'll go to gay places—be admired by men, envied by women" promised the Curvy Girl ad, which never mentioned what method you'd get for your money: an ointment, a lotion? a wish and a prayer? "I have gained three inches in 28 days" went the testimonials for Sabrina Cream (all strangely anonymous). The rather racy -sounding Lady Godiva Cream promised an eye-popping four -inch gain in 28 days along with "admiration, popularity, and affection."

At least five Sydney mail-order companies were offering the three-inches-in-28-days cream during the 1960s. One can only presume that if it worked, Sabrina, Babs O'Rourke, Paula Rae, and her cohorts would still be household names. Or were they just the same person with different post-office boxes? And were they really women? Or just weaselly men in grubby offices, getting cigar ash in their bourbon and signing themselves "Babs"?

These days Sabrina Creams have pretendy French and almost scientific names: *galbeor harmonie* (*galber* is French for "to shape or curve"), *gel multi-tenseur buste* (breast shape and firmness), and the simply stupid "bust modelling" and "contouring." This is because it's illegal to advertise something silly like "will add three inches."

No cream or lotion in the world will firm or shape or enlarge or reduce your breasts. (In previous decades protein drinks were sold which just put on weight everywhere, including the bust.) The companies claim that taut, healthy skin helps prevent sagging and that all these creams moisturise and tighten the skin. So all

a "bust-firming" gel might (*might*) do is simply tighten up the *skin* very temporarily, as a mud pack or egg white would do. And they cost a lot more than mud.

The ads—regurgitated by beauty pages as "new" information on a product—are the usual faffing on about firming plant proteins and vitamin A and hop extracts, collagen and moisturisers. One magazine, in writing about these creams under the headline "Cultivating Curves" (a big lie), quoted the founder and president of Clarins, Jacques Courtin-Clarins, as calling the skin a "natural bra" because of its "vital role in shaping the bust." This is a truly astonishing piece of stupidity. I suppose legs are nature's thigh boots and the butt is a natural pair of undies? Go and have a good lie-down, Jacques.

My favourite advertised way of changing your breasts is the cassette tape called *Natural Breast Enlargement*. You listen to the tapes for three months to overcome your problems with maximum breast development supposedly caused by trauma dur - ing puberty. (And excuse me, but who doesn't have trauma during puberty?! Which planet have they been sent to?)

It costs about $30 and tells you stuff like: "Your breasts

94

WONDER BRA   WONDER PANTS

become whatever they're willed to be. You are the authority over your breasts. You can do it. You are a winner . . . You forgive yourself for not developing to your fullest. Large, full breasts make you feel satisfied, fulfilled and vital... Your breasts grow like ripening fruit. They're warm and they're growing. . . there is a permanent tightness and firmness." And may I just add, "Liar, liar, pants on fire"?

Bras In the 1920s bras flattened out the breasts. In the 1950s they had padded bras called "falsies" or stuffed hankies down there. Now we have "dream bras" and "wonder bras" instead, which are really just...well falsies: up to $30 a bra. The "wonder bra" (what next, "wonder pants" with false bulges for men?) has most of the padding underneath the breast, pushing it up into an unnatural cleavage.

> I hate my breasts as they are very big and very uncomfortable. Difficult to buy clothes. But girls are always complaining about not having enough. I'd prefer small ones any day.
>
> Lois, 22

The media play along. "Headlines declaring 'The bust is back' have sent lingerie companies into manufacturing overdrive as they respond to the growing demand from customers for underwear that looks anything but beige," blatted one newspaper fashion page. But that's the wrong way round. The lingerie manufacturers buy advertising space, send out glossy pictures, put out press releases and advertise, and *hence* the headlines "The bust is back" (where did it go?). And Australian *Vogue* magazine has been even worse. "Small Breasts Are

Back: Making the Most of Them," its front cover shrieked in 1993, sending us all scurrying to the closet to see if our old small breasts were there waiting to be taken for a spin.

Vogue went on about how to "improve the look of the *décolletage*" (the area between the breasts) by exfoliation.

"Unfortunately, there are few advised surgical treatments to correct this highly vulnerable area of the body." What a vile notion. Dermabrasion and chemical peels were described as an option, despite a warning by dermatologists that the area is the most prone to scarring on the entire body.

"Well, thank God for makeup," prattles a witless *Vogue*. "Some brown shading between the breasts to add the effect of cleavage and a veil of powder such as Clinique's Superpowder all over the *décolletage* and neck" (just don't shake your boobs near any kryptonite). *Vogue*'s article on *décolletage* mentioned no fewer than 12 specific cosmetic products recommended for the breast area.

> My breasts are too pointy.
>
> Lindy, 15

Sales of one particular padded bra, with the pads underneath to push up the breasts, were said to be (like the breasts) alarmingly high. One British journalist gushed (or regurgitated), "The secret of the [bra] which ensures maximum uplift and a perfect shape in plunging necklines, is attributed to its 42 components, compared with only 21 in conventional bras." No, it isn't. It's attributed to the fact that it's got a humongous great bit of false padding in it. And who decides what is a perfect shape, anyway?

Sports bras are a good idea, especially to avoid annoying bouncing, sore breasts, and tearing or stretching of tissue. The good ones, made from cotton, will temporarily flatten out the breasts and have a **T**-shaped or crossover back, echoing the 1920s bras.

Some women feel the need to wear a bra only before their period, others never. Wearing a bra will not stop breasts becoming less youthful as you get older. One Australian surgeon found that 60 of his patients stopped having chronic neck and chest pain when they stopped wearing their bras. These women had too much pressure on their bra straps and nearly half of them decided they wouldn't bother with bras any more.

Big ones These are physically uncomfortable for many girls, who find that large breasts disadvantage them as they face prejudice based on appearance and ignorance similar to racism. Many girls and women with large breasts find they are rarely looked in the face by new acquaintances. "Hey, my face is up here," some of them say. Sometimes the teasing at school is agonising. The best revenge a large-breasted girl can have is not to give in to any stereotypes and to be proudly herself. Friends should be enlisted against the idiots wherever possible. (More hints in the body police section, page 213.) Large breasts which cause back problems can be reduced with surgery. Patients should find out from their doctor whether they will lose any nipple sensation or the ability to breastfeed after the operation.

Comedian Anita Wise says, "A lot of guys think the larger a woman's breasts are, the less intelligent she is...I think the larger the woman's breasts are, the less intelligent the men become."

> As I am constantly reminded, I have my grandmother's shape, short, broad hips and shoulders and a thicker waist than some. Where the big bust came from family records don't tell em. At school I was constantly teased; at least every dau someone would make a comment. It got to the point I couldn't look at myself without feeling sick. Guys were a problem too, chasing me for the wrong reasons. It's nice to be kissed at the movies instead of groped.
>
> Jade, 19

Further information

The National Cancer Institute and American Cancer Society will send you free information about breast self-examination, lumps, and cancer. See the list at the end of the book also.

If you have been diagnosed with cancer, find a support group and seek advice from women who have been through it by contacting the women's health network in your state. See the list at the end of the book.

A number of organizations work against pesticides and toxic chemicals in our environment. See that list at the end of the book.

Do I have normal thighs?

Are your thighs ruining your love life? So, you last had a date when bubble skirts were in fashion and your most recent human contact was an old-age pensioner falling on you in the bus? Could your thighs be to blame?

Could it be that Mr. Right passed you in the street only yesterday and was about to sweep you off your feet, shower you with rose petals, and canter about on a big white horse until you considered calling the ASPCA, but just as he was on the point of handing over his heart and his credit cards and insisting that he couldn't go on without you, he noticed that you had thin, taut thighs?

"Dang," muttered Mr. Right as he strode away, his ripply bits, well, rippling and the cashmere overcoat you could have borrowed swirling around him in a tragic way. "If only that woman had thighs like the girls in the Rubens paintings, I would have been her slave for the rest of my life, and always left the toilet seat down and everything."

Well I'm sorry, but it's far-fetched. When a man is feeling frisky he does not think to himself: "Good Lord! That woman's thighs do not look like the legs of a 12-year-old fashion model! I shall vow never to love her physically!"

No, by the stage of things when a man is feeling your thighs, he is more likely to have disengaged the thinking part of his brain entirely, which is why you might like to have a condom handy. The warm, soft skin on the inside of a woman's thigh—whether plump or thin— is liable to be driving him wild with desire. Honest.

If, at this point, you are thinking to yourself, "Oh my God, he's thinking that my thighs aren't perfect so I'll just tense them up to feign a bit of muscle tone," you will not be entering into the spirit of this crazed lust thing. And I'm sorry, but crazed lust beats jogging almost any way you look at it.

Worrying about being well groomed and svelte in the middle of sex (or if you don't have sex, substitute being at the pool or beach with friends) is not conducive to having a good time. It is difficult to achieve orgasm or perfect the butterfly stroke while trying to repair one's mascara and blending three lipsticks for shading purposes. (Well, I *hear* it's difficult.)

Some women have become expert at drawing attention away from their thighs. Dangling from the chandelier clad only in a dab of whipped cream and shouting, "Come over here, big boy!" is popular. So is shouting, "Look! Over there! A violent football match!" when removing the lower half of one's clothes.

Which only goes to prove that if you are one of these tortured souls, it is not your thighs ruining your love life but your self-esteem problem. So we're just going to get this out in the open, *right now.*

@

Big thighs are okay. Anybody who tries to convince you otherwise probably stands to gain, usually financially, from making you feel hideous about your legs. If you like your thighs the way they are, or accept them as just another part of you, you're not going to spend money in trying to change them, disguise them, read about them, or buy new clothes that are supposed to make you look like a trained whippet.

The people telling you you'd look better with thinner thighs are not going to ask you out, watch a video with you, be coerced into giving you a foot massage, take you home when you're not feeling well, or laugh at your jokes. No, they just want to sell you massage treatments, breakfast cereal, weight-loss programs, laxatives, frozen "diet" meals, gym membership, magazines, and useless lotions and potions. They don't even want to meet you. It is precisely because thin thighs are not the average state of womanhood that they are held up as the ideal.

> I am always 13 pounds overweight. Call me thunderthighs. You could say I go through life constantly looking for ways to improve myself and I'm almost convinced that without my dimply thighs and droopy bottom, I wouldn't need those damn [magazine] articles.
>
> Marie, 24

If most of us had perfectly fine, thin thighs instead of perfectly fine, rounded thighs, they'd be calling us scrawny and trying to convince us to buy some products which would bulk up our legs. Which they—the advertisers—will do, if they think there's money in it.

What about those models? Hey, it's their *job* to have thin thighs. They are *paid* to have thin thighs. They are naturally thinner, and then they diet and exercise for hours every day to fit into their job description and those tiny frocks.

Now, let's try this short quiz to see how we're getting on:

The thigh quiz

1. My thighs are
(a) Those bits between my torso and my gorgeous little old kneesies
(b) Like magnets to a lover's soul
(c) A hazard to shipping

2. The world is a better place for the lasting contribution made to it by
(a) Aretha Franklin
(b) The Dalai Lama
(c) Elle Macpherson

3. You would rather spend four hours
(a) With a tireless lover and a bottle of champagne
(b) Seeing how many Mint Milanos you can eat in a row without throwing up
(c) Doing a mindless, repetitive exercise to tone your thighs

4. Cellulite is
(a) French for marketing opportunity
(b) Not a recognised medical condition
(c) Taking over your entire body

5. Your best feature is
(a) Your sparkling wit
(b) Your ability to throw your voice while drinking a glass of Ovaltine
(c) The way you can spend an entire relationship backing out of rooms so he can't see the back of your legs

6. Of the following, one is most likely to ruin your love life:
(a) Your partner has this thing for short women in chicken suits
(b) Your partner is having an affair with at least three people and all the major gender groups are covered
(c) Your thighs

7. You want to move in together but your lover hasn't seen
(a) The point
(b) *Thelma and Louise*
(c) Your legs

8. If you answered (c) to any of these questions you need
(a) A good lie-down
(b) A very cunning swimsuit indeed
(c) Counselling

Top five signs that you need to get over your thigh obsession

1. It's the third date and you're still wearing the army blanket.
2. Everyone else is swimming but you're lying on the shore with your thighs swathed in cling wrap.
3. You think thighs should not wobble.
4. Liposuction doesn't sound utterly insane to you.
5. He says "You seem to be consumed with heavy sighs tonight, my love" and you think he said "I'm leaving you podgy-legs."

Who says you've got fat thighs and why? Thighs are a major concern of women. The fearful obsession that "my thighs are too fat" is used to sell magazines. One magazine carried the cover line "Who's Got the Best and Worst Thighs in Hollywood?" Inside, photographs of celebrities accompanied an article by comedian Rita Rudner called "Hollywood Thighs," which wasn't about thighs at all but about the relentless obsession with exercise in Los Angeles.

—What exercises can I do at home to get rid of cellulite around my bum?

—Why bother? It's female. Accept yourself. Celebrate yourself—that's what's beautiful!

Graffiti in Melbourne University Union building

With it the magazine ran photos of women with "truly great thighs" and "thunderthighs," none of whom was mentioned in Ms. Rudner's article. "Great" thigh owners included Madonna, who exercises for up to five hours a day, and models Naomi Campbell and Cindy Crawford, who are built thin and also exercise more than any sensible person would have time for.

The "thunderthighs" owners included Paula Abdul (a dancer!), Whitney Houston (who I'm pretty sure was photographed at a time not unadjacent to a pregnancy), and the Duchess of York, who does not, to my knowledge, live in Los Angeles, but her skirt blew up when a photographer was around. This is pure bitchiness, which is presumably supposed to make readers with normal, curvy thighs feel good that celebrities have similar ones. But it's all under the big banner of "thunderthighs": hardly a soothing definition of perfectly normal legs.

The next issue of the magazine had a cover line proclaiming that some men love "fat thighs." In the article, the man who wrote it did not call thighs "fat" at all. He didn't even think they were. W as this the magazine's definition: if not thin, then it must be fat? I asked an editor at the magazine why the word "fat" was used on the cover but not inside. She looked at me as if I were supremely stupid. "Because it sells magazines," she said. Women who think they have fat thighs will buy the magazine to read about which men like "fat" thighs but their thighs are still defined as "fat" when they are perfectly normal. (There is a definite definition problem here.)

But perhaps things are improving. Previously, another magazine had trumpeted in a cover line that it had photos of the supermodels "who used to be fat."

Of course, they didn't use to be "fat" at all, as the article pointed out. They had simply lost more

> I hate my thighs.
>
> Anonymous
>
> Because of roller skating I have big muscly legs and I used to hate that about my legs because it made the top of them look fat, but I have found out guys actually like that.
>
> Romany, 18

weight from their already underweight frames. When taken to task by a reader's letter for this ("How can we accept the way we are, reading magazine articles like these?") the magazine apologised, pleading irony.

"We're sorry!" the editor wrote on the letters page. "You misunderstood our use of the word fat. Our point was that these models could never and should never have been considered fat, yet with this trend towards 'superwaifs,' even already slim models are starving themselves into super-skinniness."

> Well the bits I don't like about myself would be my thighs but that comes with being a female.
>
> Karen, 14

In the same issue, the magazine gave valuable space to publicising a call to women to write to me if they wanted to contribute to this book about body image.

So the magazines are trying to help within the bounds of what they know will boost sales and keep their advertisers happy. Magazines will not change cover lines, including the word "fat," when they know it will sell more copies.

But magazines are not vehicles of social change, they are commercial ventures. We cannot wait for magazines to independently show a lead when it is not rewarded by sales. But we can read them more selectively and more critically. Read the magazines you like but don't take everything they say as gospel. When you see the word "fat" on the cover of a magazine, it's not necessarily accurate or relevant to your body—it's a sales tool. You do not have to accept that definition of your thighs or of yourself.

> A whole group of us girls walked into math class and the guys kept saying "thunderthighs" to one of my friends. This destroyed all her self-confidence and she told me that she cries herself to sleep every night.
>
> Daisy, 14

The great cellulite scam Cellulite is the name given to the dimply-looking fat deposits found on the thighs or legs of almost all women. It's not a name recognised by the medical profession, but it's sure as hell a "condition," "affliction," or "problem" according to the cosmetics industry. On the latest available figures, American women spend $130 million a year on cellulite creams, lotions, and "treatments."

A professor of internal medicine says, "If you're prone to getting it, cellulite will show up no matter how hard you exercise." A New York plastic surgeon says cellulite is hereditary and more common in women who have dramatic weight reductions.

A spokesperson for the Food and Drug Administration says some creams can reduce the signs of cellulite or improve the appearance by temporarily tightening the skin. You would get the exact same effect with glue or egg white. The difference made by the creams is barely visible, or invisible, but the skin feels   tighter.

Perhaps the most damning news comes from a clinical assistant professor at an American medical school who exposed the fraud of expensive rubbing devices, mitts, and creams. Stimulating the skin by scrubbing, he says, will increase the circulation and make the skin look smoother because it is causing the skin to swell up. All that happens is *low-level bruising and swelling*.

> Don't think that thin people don't have cellulite —we do!
>
> Catherine, 17

"People who fall for these creams misunderstand the structure of their bodies," says another New York plastic surgeon. "There's no cream in the world that will restore elasticity to your skin." She adds that lotions and creams cannot eliminate toxins, break up body fat, or have a diuretic effect.

Let's get something clear. *All* grown-up women have fat on their thighs. This does not make them "fat thighs," or too fat.

Marie Claire, an English and French magazine, has completely lost the plot about thighs. After all, the cellulite scam was invented in France, where they are allowed to sell a cream marketed as a Quick Slimming Complexe—called Body Contour Cream elsewhere—with fat- and cellulite-reducing properties. In Australia and the United States such a "fat-melting" claim would have to be proved with tests and studies, so the advertising in those countries does not make the same claims. *Marie Claire* magazine awarded it Best Cream of the Year in a vote by European beauty editors.

Another *Marie Claire* article about cellulite epitomises the very worst of "beauty reporting." Its report read: "Between the ages of fifteen and 50, up to 80 percent of women are susceptible to cellulite, according to shape specialists Elancyl."

Shape specialists? What's a shape specialist? In this case it's a cosmetics company that makes a fortune out of selling cellulite "treatments." Shape specialists, if you don't mind me saying, my ass.

Cellulite tends to accumulate, says the company, before menopause, in contraceptive pill users, during pregnancy, in times of stress, during emotional trauma, in smokers, and in people who don't exercise a lot. It makes perfect sense if you recognise that cellulite is really normal deposits of padding that all women—even thin women—have (menopause, smoking, and stress aside).

Another magazine listed "treatments" including lying in sand for 30 minutes at a time, saunas, a friction rub (well, we know what that does), marine algae wraps, aromatherapy, reflexology, an entire body exfoliation, diet, exercise, not getting tense, electrodes attached to "the parts of the body needing treatment" to stimulate muscles instead of exercising (eek!), vibration machines, herbal oils, being attached to a thermal heat machine, aerobics, step aerobics, weightlifting, and lotions (naming all the cosmetics companies' major products) with ingredients including "liposomes," "non-ionic microspheres," "marine life derivatives," "kaolin" (which is ordinary clay), "centella asiatica," "micro-reservoirs of collagen," unspecified "key ingredients," and sunflower oil.

Then the magazine listed seven separate thigh moisturisers all by cosmetic company and trade name. Just another ad.

"It may be worth investing in Shiseido's Body Exfoliating Scrub [$23] too. Active plant extracts such as the circulatory aid butcher's broom, as well as ivy and caffeine (which both have contouring properties) are common anti-cellulite ingredients; sometimes they are combined with synthetic chemicals to make their fat-busting powers more potent," the magazine continued shamelessly. Oo-er.

Let's just examine that statement like the new detectives we are. Will we be bamboozled by the pseudo-science? What's an active plant extract anyway—something from a potted plant that goes jogging? It's just jargon.

And the circulatory aids—well, anything is a circulatory aid if you're vigorously rubbing it in and scrubbing; do that anywhere on your skin without a product and you'll get an improvement in circulation as blood rushes to the surface. In fact, German lederhosen dances in which you slap your thighs will probably have the same effect, although you'd have to listen to polka music.

And as for the phrase "fat-busting," it sounds like an ad, is hardly scientific, and is not backed up by any evidence. In fact, it is a slogan and nothing more.

We have been conned. The multimillion-dollar cosmetics companies, aided by women's magazines who have swallowed their propaganda hook, line, and sinker, are trying to convince us our natural curves and padding are "unsightly."

My friend Stephanie was told at a Clarins counter that there was "nothing worse than cellulite." "How about nuclear war?" she replied. The saleswoman looked sceptical.

Stretch marks When an area of the body gets bigger or smaller quickly—like when you develop bigger hips, breasts, and thighs at puberty—it often leaves stretch marks.

> I have so many stretch marks.
>
> Sally-Anne, 17

This also happens with rapid weight gain and loss, so it's common among dieters. And lots of pregnant women get stretch marks on their tummy, bottom, and legs as everything gets bigger in readiness for the baby.

Like "cellulite" and body shape, a tendency to stretch marks is hereditary. This is not an excuse to go and shout at your parents. As if you need one.

Some doctors and herbalists say that people deficient in zinc and vitamin B6 are more prone to the marks, and vitamin E tablets and creams are recommended by some women who have used them during pregnancy. But other dermatologists say that there is usually only a tiny amount of vitamin E in a lotion and it's not certain it can penetrate the skin.

The marks are often in the form of red or purple lines, but over time, they will fade to a shimmer and become hardly noticeable unless you're inspecting yourself closely with a magnifying glass or fretting about it.

> I have stretch marks on my hips, thighs, and butt. I hate them but I am slowly getting used to them cos they are fading.
>
> Maeve, 15

By the time we're all grown up, almost all women have them, many without ever noticing. Others hide, wearing shorts and refusing to go swimming and missing out on a feeling of freedom and fun.

Do I have normal periods?

Visit from a friend To understand periods, you need to understand that a woman's life is like a cycle (although not very much like a unicycle) and that after puberty, usually in our early teens, we start having a monthly menstrual cycle. This goes on until menopause in middle age.

Every month one or the other ovary releases an egg, which if fertilised by sperm will become an embryo—the start of a baby. (We can stop this from happening by not losing our minds with lust without using some form of contraception.)

Menstruating, or a period, or friend, or being "on the rag" is what happens when the body realises you haven't fertilised the nice egg it made for you and the egg and the extra thickening on the inside of your womb—where an embryo would have grown—are expelled through "bleeding."

The amount of the average bleed is only 1.5 fluid ounces over two to seven days, although it often seems to be more. Periods can start from the age of 10 to 17-ish and visit regularly until you're between 45 and 55. All these statistics vary widely from woman to woman and there is a wide variation of "normal."

Anything which changes radically for the woman may be abnormal for her, like suddenly getting heavy periods, or a shorter cycle each time. A change for just one cycle can usually be ignored.

If you haven't ovulated (released the egg) you can still get a period. Some people miss a few periods here and there, others get one every 28 days regular as anything, and some people have one every three months or three weeks: all these can be "normal."

Many religions and cultures held or even still hold that menstruation is a taboo. Women are banned from churches and kitchens during their period. This is because people who don't fully understand the process think it is unclean and bizarre. Given that it will happen to more than half the population during most of their lives, this kind of attitude is pretty pathetic.

The embarrassment extends to coy advertising. Some of you may be wondering why they advertise pads and tampons by putting blue ink on them. So are the rest of us. The only person who ever had a blue period was Picasso. Don't be embarrassed about your period. (Unless it's blue.)

Here are some things you can do SIMULTANEOUSLY with having your period (but only if you really want to): have sex, swim, have showers or baths, drive a large passenger train, and dance. Although I wouldn't recommend trying to drive a passenger train and dance simultaneously. (I be that party pooper.)

This is not to say that when your period first happens it isn't amazing and special and kind of scary, even if you've been warned about it. It's part of becoming a woman. And yes, it is natural that you can smell the blood after it has contact with the air. It is very unlikely that anyone else can, although dogs, with their incredibly acute, inhuman sense of smell, will often try and put their noses in your crotch at that time of the month. Which is one reason why you should only cultivate friendships with people who have short dogs.

⊚

Menstrual diary Because your period is an indication of whether or not you are pregnant, as well as general health, and sometimes a mood predictor, it's a good idea to keep a record of it. Include details and dates of any changes in the colour (what kind of red or brown), amount, or consistency of the blood (and it's not just blood—bits of uterine-lining tissue get expelled in the natural process), any pre-menstrual symptoms, the nature and times of any pain, and, once you've established a pattern, when the next period is likely.

This can be very helpful to you and your health-care practitioner—and those close to you, who can make plans to go interstate whenever you're pre-menstrual. Here's a calendar you can cut out or photocopy and keep somewhere you'll use it.

Don't be surprised if you find that your period ends up synchronised with the other women you live, work, or study

Your Menstrual Calendar

Keep track of the little euphemism through the year. Easy to find out how regular you are, or if your period is late. Circle each day of your period throughout the year and watch your pattern emerge. This chart should not be used for contraception unless you want to have vast quantities of babies. If you need contraception, use condoms instead.

Jan 1	29	26	25	21	18	15	13	9	5	3	31	27	25
2	30	27	26	22	19	16	14	10	6	4	Nov	28	26
3	31	28	27	23	20	17	15	11	7	5	1	29	27
4	Feb 1	Mar	28	24	21	18	16	12	8	6	2	30	28
5	2	1	29	25	22	19	17	13	9	7	3	Dec 1	29
6	3	2	30	26	23	20	18	14	10	8	4	2	30
7	4	3	31	27	24	21	19	15	11	9	5	3	31
8	5	4	Apr	28	25	22	20	16	12	10	6	4	Jan 1
9	6	5	1	29	26	23	21	17	13	11	7	5	2
10	7	6	2	30	27	24	22	18	14	12	8	6	3
11	8	7	3	May	28	25	23	19	15	13	9	7	4
12	9	8	4	1	29	26	24	20	16	14	10	8	5
13	10	9	5	2	30	27	25	21	17	15	11	9	6
14	11	10	6	3	31	28	26	22	18	16	12	10	7
15	12	11	7	4	Jun 1	29	27	23	19	17	13	11	8
16	13	12	8	5	2	30	28	24	20	18	14	12	9
17	14	13	9	6	3	Jul 1	29	25	21	19	15	13	10
18	15	14	10	7	4	2	30	26	22	20	16	14	11
19	16	15	11	8	5	3	31	27	23	21	17	15	12
20	17	16	12	9	6	4	Aug	28	24	22	18	16	13
21	18	17	13	10	7	5	1	29	25	23	19	17	14
22	19	18	14	11	8	6	2	30	26	24	20	18	15
23	20	19	15	12	9	7	3	31	27	25	21	19	16
24	21	20	16	13	10	8	4	Sep	28	26	22	20	17
25	22	21	17	14	11	9	5	1	29	27	23	21	18
26	23	22	18	15	12	10	6	2	30	28	24	22	19
27	24	23	19	16	13	11	7	3	Oct 1	29	25	23	20
28	25	24	20	17	14	12	8	4	2	30	26	24	21

This menstrual calendar is in lines of 28 days, the "average" time between periods. But some modern girls get a period every 16 days or every couple of months.

with. Nobody is quite sure why this happens, although they suspect some sort of unconscious armpit sniffing. Personally, I think it's a kind of subconscious etiquette. "Let's get this PMS stuff over and done with all at once. Behold the bite marks on the furniture! Express an opinion if ye dare! Cower in terror, ye visitors to the house of HELL!"

@

Pre-menstrual syndrome (PMS) Pre-menstrual symptoms include fluid retention that results in bigger, tighter, and sorer breasts, bloated stomach, low self-esteem, increased weight everywhere, pimples usually before but sometimes also during and/ or after the period, moodiness, clumsiness, back pain, leg pain, being furious, loss of concentration abilities, depression, a bizarrely determined need for chocolate, confusion, and general unspecific crabbiness and tears. Also insomnia, headaches, and, more rarely, manic behaviour like cleaning out the inside of the fridge even though it isn't your turn.

All of this has do with the complex relationship between the mysterious HORMONES, estrogen and progesterone. More research into the syndrome (or syndromes) is needed. Some doctors still will not acknowledge its existence because it is so hard to measure. Studies have shown that some women are prone to extreme behavior just before their period—for example, eating a block of chocolate approximately the size of Mount Rushmore.

One idea is to flag your pre-menstrual days to your family or housemates by hanging a red scarf or flag (or bedspread, if things are really tough) on the calendar or on the fridge for the duration. Then when they say, "Good morning!" and you bark, "Start that kind of talk with me and I'll run you through with a bayonet!" they can just ignore you instead of calling the police. On the other hand, maybe they should have called the police.

Take your menstrual diary to a doctor or natural healer who can help you decide what is best for your symptoms. You may have to rifle the neighbourhood for the right "health professional"— ask around. Natural healers and doctors often suggest evening primrose oil capsules, along with vitamin B6 in doses larger than usually recommended. Both these things are cheaper in bulk at the supermarket than at health food shops. Natural healers are likely to ask you many questions, aiming to prescribe treatments best suited to your individual needs. The times to take tablets (just during pre-menstrual time or all month) will vary between women.

Diuretics, which make you pee a lot and lose the fluid retention, may also be prescribed. Chemical ones can strip the body of potassium and magnesium, and herbal ones such as celery juice or celery and juniper herbal tablets may work less dramatically. Because unripe juniper berries may cause kidney problems, you should follow the packet instructions and not use the tablets continuously for more than two months. They should not be used by people with kidney disease. Dandelion leaf tea is good and contains plenty of potassium and magnesium. (Personally I think it tastes like boiled grass clippings.) Beware of taking too many diuretics, which will dehydrate your body.

Also, not being stressed can help as the uterus spasms will not be so painful. Stress can alter the state of our hormones and bring on an imbalance. This is why some people swear by yoga, massage, exercise, and other relaxation methods.

Other medications include anti-inflammatory drugs; chamomile, raspberry leaf, peppermint, fresh ginger, and red clover teas; acupuncture; calcium tablets; aspirin; essential fatty acids other than primrose oil; minerals; and progesterone therapy.

PMS sufferers should eat between meals! And have little snacks often in the days before their period. Eating fruit, raw veggies, nuts, or soy milk will keep up protein and cut excessive, yo-yoing blood-sugar levels. This will stave off the chocolate cravings, too. Cut down on salt, which aids fluid retention; caffeine, which will make you wired; and sugar, which can spiral you into more sugar cravings. Tobacco and alcohol just confuse the situation (as is their wont).

It never arrived There are several reasons for not getting your period including pregnancy, breastfeeding, ill-health perhaps due to drugs, severe physical or psychological stress, overexercise, and poor nutrition.

If you have not started having periods by the age of 17 see a doctor or go to a family-planning clinic. But don't panic—and remember, everyone is different. If you miss two periods in your usual cycle, it should be checked out.

The scientific "Hottie"

Period pain This is really common. "Cramps" are simply that—often just before or on the first day of the period spasms of the uterus help expel the blood.

The trick is not to put up with very bad pain, or mask it with very strong painkillers or anti-spasm drugs. It is your body telling you there is something wrong and not "a woman's lot" that must be endured. Do not put up with pain which interferes with your lifestyle and cannot be controlled by recommended doses of low-level painkillers. This pain may include vomiting, nausea, aching or stabbing pains before, during, and after a period, violent cramps, or similarly awful pains at ovulation.

Find a sympathetic doctor and/or natural healer and make them earn your money. If your doctor tells you the pain is normal or neurotic behaviour, or something that women must put up with, lurch across the desk with your eyes rolling and attempt to strangle him or her, screaming politely, "Is this NORMAL?!"

Trust your instincts and insist on a referral to a menstruation specialist. You may be easily relieved of your pain by a course of tablets, or find that you have a treatable menstrual disorder such as endometriosis, in which some blood doesn't leave the body (it gets absorbed) because it's from functioning endometrial tissue (like the lining of the uterus) that has grown in places it shouldn't be. Or pelvic inflammatory disease, in which the tubes, the ovaries, the tubes and ovaries, and/or the uterus become infected. If PID and endometriosis are not treated, they may cause terrible pain and infertility later on.

As for your "average" cramps—herbal remedies, heat (such as a hot-water bottle, known by its scientific name, the "hottie"), swimming, and yoga exercises have helped some women to banish period pain.

◎

Pads Natural therapists and some doctors recommend that you use pads whenever possible. Pads allow for a more natural flow.

◎

Tampons Always use the lowest absorbency for your needs and try to use pads whenever possible. Tampons can absorb natural moisture as well as blood in the vagina, so at least use pads at night during your period. If your tampon is hard to remove, there's not enough fluid to make it necessary, so swap to a light pad. Tampons should not be left in for more than six hours and never overnight.

Using tampons for the first time will not mean that you are no longer a virgin. Don't force anything that hurts. Follow the instructions in the packet and don't be shy of gently stretching your vagina, over time, with your (clean) fingers. (Lock the door first!)

Further reading

The best book about what happens to your body is *The New Our Bodies Ourselves*, by the Boston Women's Health Book Collective (New York: Touchstone Books, 1992). If you can't afford it, hassle your library until it gets a copy.

Women's health centres and Planned Parenthood clinics should have specific pamphlets on menstruation.

Do I have normal skin?

Acne and pimples Experts disagree about exactly what causes all pimples. (It makes you wonder why we bother having experts, really.) Hormones definitely play the major part, which is why you might get pimples before your period. Almost all experts now say eating four blocks of chocolate has nothing to do with pimples. Only a handful still say that food is a factor, but we have locked them all in the broom closet.

You can probably work out whether food, stress, smoking, and hormone cycles and irregularities affect your skin by keeping track of them and any subsequent mad pimplefest your skin responds with.

You can keep pimples down to a dull roar by washing carefully with soap and water as often as you need, to cut down the oiliness in your skin. I know everybody says it, but don't touch pimples because it can cause infection which may result in scarring. Get out of the habit of resting your chin in the palm of your hand, for example. Try not to squeeze pimples, especially if they're not ready, because this can leave bruising and even scars.

Acne creams from the pharmacist can abrade the skin, making it peel away. Be careful you don't use too much. Very hard drying agents such as alcohol and peroxide can also cause nasty-looking skin peeling around a pimple.

The major problem, feral hormones, is very common during adolescence and not unknown thereafter. At puberty, hormones enlarge the glands and get them to produce more oil. This can continue throughout your life, particularly before a period, or while taking contraceptive pills. A hormone imbalance can be helped by a doctor or herbalist.

> I used to get called names like "space face crater," "Pizza Hut," "spotty," and more. This made me feel extremely sad, distressed, and very hurt. I kept myself as healthy as possible and did the right things but my skin is still rough and has open pores. People say I'm pretty anyway. I feel awful, though. When I look at the models in magazines I feel cheated.
>
> Anonymous

Some natural therapists believe that toxins such as smoke, alcohol, many drugs including prescribed and illegal, anaesthetics, and environmental poisoning may cause pimples as the body tries every way it can to get rid of them. Most dermatologists disagree.

All dermatologists *do* agree that despite the rumour, drinking more water will have *no effect* on your skin.

Eighty percent of people get pimples and there's a plan to send the rest to another planet as soon as we have the technology. For most people, the pimple stage passes. If you are concerned, you can get a referral to a dermatologist from your local physician. Make sure that any drug treatment is fully explained to you, including risks and side effects.

Steer clear of chemical skin peels. That's your top layers of skin they're ripping off your face. Peels should be done only by a qualified dermatologist—if you're really determined to submit yourself to it.

By the way, you can squeeze blackheads, but no known product has been invented that will change the size of your pores and stop them filling up again. Everybody has blackheads.

◎

Tanning Do you want the bad news first or the good news first? We might as well get right in amongst it: skin cancer. The United States has one of the highest rates in the world. It can kill you if it can kill 9,200 Americans a year, at last count. This means any mole or lump or warty thing on your body should be checked and then rechecked by a doctor if you detect *any* changes in feel or appearance. Some skin marks are harmless and very common, such as freckles, skin tags, moles, and beauty marks and spots. Melanomas (the most nasty skin cancers—they metastasise) usually start as flat, coloured spots. The colour may begin as, or develop to, white, red, pink, light brown, dark brown, or black.

Most sun experts agree that the more sunburns you have had, the more likely you are to get skin cancer.

The National Cancer Institute recommends staying out of the sun between 10 A.M. and 2 P.M., or 11 A.M. and 3 P.M. during daylight saving time. They'd like you to have a broad-brimmed hat that casts a solid shade all around (not a baseball cap); use a sunscreen not less than SPF 15, applied at least 15 minutes before you are in the sun, and every two hours

> My friends just go to the beach and lie there all day with their coconut oil, browning up nicely in the sun. All the girls in the magazines are brown while I sit there, packing on the SPF 15 and trying to cover up all my exposed skin. I stay white and have a few more freckles for the collection.
>
> Teresa, 21

(more if you've been in the water), hang out in the shade where possible, and wear sunglasses to American National Standard Z80.3 so your eyeballs don't get roasted (or something to do with ultra-violet ray damage).

The biggest danger period is the middle of the day at any time and especially from May to September, when UV (ultraviolet) radiation is 10 to 20 times stronger than it is the rest of the year. But don't forget that surfaces like concrete and snow can throw up massive UV reflections and burn you.

When applying sunscreen, don't forget your fiddly bits such as lips, ears, backs of the knees, toes, elbows, and the back of your neck. The upper back, which is difficult to reach by yourself, is a common place for melanoma skin cancers.

◎

Fake tans Who was that giant carrot? That was me in a fake tan. The sales of fake tanning creams have risen with the awareness of the dangers of real tans. No models will tan. All of them use fake ones if required for a job.

Fake tans are scary for many reasons. One, we don't know their long-term effects. Two, they're expensive and they only last a few days. Some wash off in water. Three, they induce a false sense of security but offer no protection against real sunburn. Four, they continue the idea that a tan is fashionable, which keeps idiots out there every summer frying themselves silly. Five, they can stain clothes and furniture, and six, they can make you look like a giant carrot with brown palms.

Spooky time: solariums are where tans are produced by sun lamps and sun beds. The National Cancer Institute is rabidly opposed to them and here's why. Most solariums claim their fluorescent tubes emit only UVA ultraviolet radiation rays but many also emit

UVB rays. Until recently it was thought that UVA rays were harmless, but now we know they cause premature wrinkling. Some evidence also links them with skin cancers.

UVB rays are the most likely to cause sunburn and skin damage leading to skin cancer . UVB rays are dangerous to the eyes. Some drugs and cosmetics can increase a person's vulnerability to ultraviolet rays, including contraceptive pills, antibiotics, and tranquillizers. To remember which is which, think of it this way: UVB for burn and UVA for ageing.

Lots of people think they look healthier with a tan, hence the fake-tan trend, which will be encouraged and perpetuated by images of tanned models in fashion magazines that take much of their revenue from the cosmetic companies selling fake tans. Many magazine stories have heartily recommended—even insisted on—fake tans, which their manufacturers would rather call (inaccurately) self-tans.

@

Bleaching Dangerous lightening and bleaching creams are available all over the world and are common and popular in European, American, Asian, African, Caribbean, and other countries where people with darker skin are discriminated against, and where an Anglo-Saxon ideal of beauty and wealth is advertised or glorified. Bleaching and lightening chemicals can cause burns, premature ageing, and patchy, mottled effects. And anyway, Indian, Asian, Aboriginal, African, and Islander skins are beautiful just the way they are.

Do I have normal smells?

Sweating Everybody sweats. As a matter of fact, most of us sweat about $2\frac{1}{2}$ pints of sweat each 24 hours, without exercise. With exercise we become dripping soggy things, losing up to a quart an hour.

This is because we each have about 3 million sweat glands all over the body. (What was that noise? That was my mind boggling.) Tight clothes and most unnatural fabrics don't allow the sweat to evaporate, which makes for a stickier feeling.

⊚

Armpits Deodorants and antiperspirants each work in different ways. Antiperspirants are made from aluminum. This shrinks pores and reduces the amount of sweat able to escape from the body. Antiperspirants are more likely to cause allergies and irritations than are deodorants, which kill bacteria, the element in sweat which causes it to smell. Deodorants do not interfere with the natural process of sweating.

A natural deodorising crystal has been developed which has no chemicals or perfumes and can be rubbed under your armpits. The small deoderant crystal, used every day, will last up to a year!

Some people don't use deodorant or antiperspirant at all, preferring to wash regularly. Because we all sweat differently, some people who use deodorant products may sweat more than somebody with *au naturel* pits.

Body odour from the armpits and genital areas is normal. The body produces chemical attractants from these areas to arouse sexual partners. While some people scrub off the odours or douse themselves in perfumes to cover the smells, scientists are desperate to discover how to bottle the scents, known as pheromones, so they can sell it as perfume!

As for shaving, generally women in the United States do, women in Europe don't. Most Australian women are influenced by what their friends do and by habit. Just don't let anyone tell you armpit hair is weird or gross or unusual. Millions of women have free-range armpits.

⊚

The parts in your pants It is very important never to put deodorant or perfume, or any kind of douche or spray, up into the vagina or onto the genital area. Your apparatus is self-cleaning on the inside and you can do the rest yourself every day on the outside bits with soap and water and a good rinse. The chemicals in "feminine hygiene" products can throw out the natural balance of the yeasts and friendly bacteria in your vagina and many people get rashes from using these on such sensitive skin. Yowww.

Do I have normal teeth?

Tooth wrangling Think carefully before considering braces. Are they intended to correct a problem with chewing? Because your teeth will last longer if they're not crowding each other out? Because you know it's what you want? Is it a teeny tiny overbite nobody else really notices? Is having them something you may regret later, or have you really thought it through and discussed it with friends and family? Are you doing it just because the dentist says you should, and your parents assume you want it? Are you just temporarily sensitive about your teeth because of a comment from a dork who was trying to make himself feel superior? Could we perhaps put out a contract on the dork instead?

When considering "bonding" (sounds like what men do on wilderness/percussion camping holidays) to fill a gap between teeth or cover a chip, think about the unique character you might erase from your face. Be aware that the bond itself is more vulnerable to chipping than tooth enamel and find out which foods might stain the bonding materials. Also remember that a chipped tooth may be more vulnerable to decay, and that bonding may stop you feeling self-conscious about smiling. Check whether your bonding is reversible. And be prepared for people not to notice. As in, "Have you changed your hairstyle or something?"

Never have teeth removed unnecessarily. The natural tooth is always better and less likely to run into trouble if you look after it.

Don't automatically agree to anything: go home and consider

your options with the help of pamphlets or photocopied explanations from the dentist's office and your own notes on prices. Remember that a purely cosmetic treatment can be put off but a long delay in treatment for a health problem in your mouth will almost certainly lead to more pain and costs later on.

Don't be talked into anything cosmetic by a smooth-talking dentist who plays on your insecurities about your smile. Some dentists have a ridiculous chart called a Smile Assessment Chart in which your teeth are rated, and your smile given a score, or even a "fail." (Patients should be able to respond with a Dentist's Personality Assessment Chart.) This is nothing but a way of getting you to spend money. It is not scientific and in my opinion you should not go back to a dentist who uses one. The American Dental Association in your area will provide free advice on choosing the right dentist.

Cosmetic surgery

Who needs it? Cosmetic surgery is not gentle. It's about cutting, slicing, gouging, grasping, pulling, blood, bruising and plastic drains left poking out of wounds to allow fluids to escape from the body after an operation. The bulk of the work is violent, unnecessary surgery on healthy people which is presented more prettily and inaccurately as "nips and tucks" or "sculpting." Somewhere along the line the bizarre, scary, degrading practice of surgery on normal women gained respectability from the media and writers such as Dr. Miriam Stoppard. She refers to the purpose of liposuction as removing "unsightly bulges such as at the top of thighs and the arms."

She advises that "with modern operations and new techniques of cosmetic surgery, it is possible to re-contour almost any part of the body if you are unhappy with the shape you've got... What you have to weigh up is the trade-off: are you the kind of woman who wants to look good in clothes, or do you wish to be free from scars when you are naked?"

Actually, Miriam, old sausage, I'm the kind of woman who doesn't want to undergo general anaesthesia unless I have no choice. I'm the kind of woman who thinks "cosmetic" surgery is only okay in the most extreme cases—breast reduction to stop back pain, for example. I'm the kind of woman who thinks that your book describing gouging and cutting out bits of arm as "simple and straightforward" is misleading and an advocacy of mutilation.

◎

Guinea pigs Women have been used as guinea pigs for cosmetic surgery since 1903 when Chicago doctor Charles Miller opened the first cosmetic surgery practice. Miller cut into his customers' bodies and inserted bits of "braided silk, bits of silk floss, particles of celluloid, vegetable ivory and several other foreign materials" according to his own account of 1926. He returned to general surgery during the Great Depression when demand for cosmetic surgery dropped away.

In the 1920s doctors removed the healthy breasts of women who could not emulate the flat-chested fashion of the day. And all in the name of profit, in the guise of helping women's self-esteem.

◎

Publicity The only recognised experts in the field are plastic surgeons, of course, and you don't hear much from them about pain (often described as "discomfort" or "problems"). Pain, especially extended pain over hours, days, and weeks, can have a terrible effect on the body and the mind in physical and psychological shock and distress. The pain, bruising, and damage done to the body by many cosmetic surgery operations are comparable to injuries sustained during a car accident.

Newspapers perpetuate the hard sell. "Give Yourself a Lift," says one headline. "Thinking about a face lift—why not go the whole hog and get a complete make-over?" the article began. "Those magnificent men with their cutting devices can snip, tuck, tighten, reduce, increase and streamline almost every part of the human body."

An unnamed surgeon quoted in the article said most of

his customers did not have operations because of vanity but because of their "deformities." He classed a big nose and small breasts as deformities, adding that a woman with small breasts "can't wear certain types of clothes. Whenever she is with other women who wear tight T-shirts or clothes and who look a bit feminine, she feels just not feminine."

The surgeon complained that GPs often sent their patients home who asked for a referral to a plastic surgeon and had to wait for another "trigger incident" to provoke a more spirited request. " For example they might have broken up with a boyfriend or separated from a husband or they are under other stresses and they feel this is one stress they want to unload." Very vulnerable people should be reassured, not cut open.

Magazines often run "before and after" photographs of surgery. The "after " photographs are usually taken once the swelling and bruising have faded. There are never "during" photos or "straight after " photos or "two years later" photos.

Amateur hour Cosmetic surgery sounds kind of attractive and scientific, but any general practitioner can call himself a cosmetic surgeon and do skin peels and collagen injections. The Complaints Unit of an Australian health department produces pamphlets about cosmetic surgery "in the public interest," advising people considering more serious surgery on how to get a competent plastic surgeon and giving information about the procedure. Pain is not mentioned. There is no pamphlet on reasons not to have surgery, or other options to consider instead of plastic surgery. Almost all the information we have on procedures comes directly from surgeons or clinics, not exactly unbiased sources.

Cosmeticians, or cosmetic doctors, or "aesthetic surgeons" may have no specialist training. The American Society of Plastic and Reconstructive Surgeons says only its "board-certified" members are properly qualified. In Australia, one woman who had a face lift at a clinic because she saw their advertisement spent $5,250 on a botched job which left her with raised, red scars, eyes that would not close for months, and asymmetrical eyelids.

Liposuction Although most surgery brochures do not mention pain, all accounts by liposuction customers do. A ustralian *Fashion Quarterly* interviewed some of them. "It hurt like hell for a month," says one, who says now she's out of proportion because fat has gathered in places it never used to—her waist and knees. "Now I'm more depressed than I was before I had liposuction, because now that escape route from fatness, which I saved for 18 months to afford, has been taken away from me." It seems the natural padding had lost its natural home. She took "mind-numbing" painkillers. "It was painful even to walk...I had liposuction to make me look thinner, but I couldn't move so I put on more weight." Another woman was left with scarring from the metal tubes stuck through her skin to break up and suck up fat cells.

Another woman, who had liposuction by an internationally renowned surgeon, had ballooned in the torso and waist. "In my

case, I think, the operation unbalanced me for a while, although I don't blame anyone else for that. It was so incredibly painful."
"If you look at some of the earlier facial liposuction devotees their faces aren't sleek—they're gaunt, skeletonised," reported the magazine. "I suffered widespread bruising and couldn't sit down for about three weeks," said another woman. "It was a disaster. I ended up using my whole year's holiday to recover."

An Australian *Mode* reporter wrote of her liposuction. She recalled feeling like a victim of her culture as she dialled the surgeon on the telephone. "Like most women, I disliked my hips and thighs. Unlike most women, I was lucky enough to have the money to do something about them." She said that her father had plump hips and her shape is genetic.

"What nobody tells you beforehand is that you're only sedated at the very last moment and you will have to face your doctor and his staff wide awake and naked." Knocked out, the customer does not hear the grinding, "gruesome sound" of the liposuction machine or see the operating team shift the body like a piece of meat, "using your bootee-covered feet as handles."

She added, "For the first 12 hours post-op you must urinate about every ten minutes, at a time when sitting down is about as comfortable as swallowing molten lead...I have a fairly high tolerance for pain, but the first few days after surgery I lay on my stomach munching Percodan. For two weeks thereafter I lumbered stiffly to work like Frankenstein, knowing that one careless bump into another human being would make me scream...

"The aching continued, only gradually diminishing, for three months... The seventh week after surgery you're supposed to be able to run. I couldn't, and neither could any of the patients I spoke to. It took ten weeks." She cited 12 reported liposuction deaths in the United States and one woman who was left with a hole in her thigh and haemorrhaging underneath the skin from knee to ankle.

"Standard liposuction," she said, "rips out the fat globules through suction and the sheer muscle power of the surgeon." Next, the reporter wants to have the bags under her eyes cut out. But she's not doing this for her man. "Two weeks before surgery I met the man I'll probably marry. He liked my hips and thighs the way they were."

Noses One clinic, which performs plastic surgery in Sydney, does nothing to reassure people about their magnificent honkers. They go so far as to recommend deviousness to avoid someone who loves you advising you against a painful, non-medical operation. "A large or deformed nose can often attract undesirable comment. Ultimately one's self-confidence can erode and personality problems may develop. The modern rhinoplasty is a simple and safe operation which readily overcomes this potential social dilemma [sic]... The fewer people you tell about your proposed operation the better. By all means discuss your operation with a close friend, they will be in a position to give you sympathetic and unbiased advice. In contrast to this, members of your family who have known you from childhood are, for emotional reasons, inclined to advise you against having any facial alterations." Oh, emotional reasons, like love. Pah. Pass the scalpel, sweetie.

@

The breast business explained By a conservative estimate, at least 2 million American women have had breast implants in the last 25 years.

Fake breasts are now made from a liquid-saline (salt) filler contained in a solid bag made from the same stuff they use for replacement heart valves. You know why? Because so many women have sued the makers of the previous breast filling, silicone, which is a close chemical relative to Silly Putty.

For years, women have told stories of hardening, lumpy breasts, silicone lumps moving up under armpits, and rupturing during mammography tests for breast cancer. Implants also make it harder to detect breast cancer.

And liquid-saline implants that are encased in a rubbery shell made of silicone (not the heart valve stuff) carry a risk of deflation and leaking.

Medical journalists predicted that the leaking of the silicone gel implants would cause immune problems. And so it came to pass. By August 1993, when *Vogue* reported it, Dow Corning admitted that tests on rats showed silicone to be a strong irritant to the immune system, but that did not mean that this could necessarily be applied to humans. Soon after, a California study found that one-

It would be WRONG to experiment on animals.... while we have WOMEN!

KAZ

third of women with implants have a measurable immune system reaction.

It is now estimated that there have been many breakages and leakages from silicone implants and that, in those women, anecdotal evidence supports disruption of the immune system. "It is well established," reported Dr. Ronald Laura in *Nature and Health* magazine, that "small amounts of silicone fluid seep from all silicone gel implants, even when they are not ruptured." Many women who have had silicone leakage have reported symptoms ranging from arthritis-like pain, swelling of the joints, skin, hands, and feet, and hair loss to lupus and other immune system diseases. The U.S. Food and Drug Administration (FDA) received more than 23,000 reports of problems with implants in 1992 and more than 19,000 in 1994.

One young woman who had breast implants at the age of 18 went through hell as they ruptured and leaked, causing pain and anxiety, and another operation to remove the bags. She still has the pain that started after the rupturing. "I feel like ripping out my spine," she said. "I want to tell girls who are thinking about implants [that] we should stay the way we're born and not have anything artificial in us."

This kind of major operation should be considered with great caution. The FDA placed a ban on silicone breast implants in April 1992, which still has not been lifted. The FDA's policy makes these implants available only through controlled clinical trials; such clinical trials are already established for reconstructive sugery, but no trials for augmentation surgery had yet begun by December 1994.

And although the results of the many studies conducted to examine the extent or damage to the body from implants have been disputed by the implant manufacturers, women have turned out in large numbers to file lawsuits against these manufacturers for injury claims. More than 25,000 women have already sought action, bringing 12,000 cases to the courts. The legal system has awarded monetary compensation to a few women who have filed civil suits for damages. These women had implants inserted on the premise that the information that the manufacturers had provided was valid. Some of the companies claimed that the bags were inert and would last a lifetime.

The Breast Implant Litigation Fund Three manufacturers, Dow Corning Corporation, Bristol Meyers–Squibb Company, and Baxter Healthcare Corporation, and their insurance companies have set up a fund which allocates $3.7 billion over 30 years for women who received a silicone gel implant or a saline-filled implant with a silicone coating. The companies have done so without admitting guilt in an effort, they say, to avoid additional litigation costs. It is the largest settlement ever negotiated in a class-action lawsuit.

The precise percentages of this total allocation have not yet been determined, but roughly $1.2 billion would be used towards compensation for women who have been diagnosed by a medical review panel as presently suffering from one of eight diseases caused by the implants; $1.9 million would be reserved for women who develop these diseases, and $635 million would be used for various services or treatments (including medical monitoring and implant removal) over a period of 30 years for women who do not have health problems. These monies will also cover compensation for those who have had breast implants rupture and those who are suffering from post-implant emotional anguish.

Compensation will be determined by age, and also type and severity of medical problem. Children of women with breast implants could be covered under this settlement if they develop health problems which are believed to be related to silicone exposure.

Critics of the settlement say that with the great numbers of women who presently have implants, the fund may be depleted by the time women who are getting the implants now develop problems in the future. There are no definite plans for what happens once all compensation money gets doled out.

What this actually means is that breast implants are bad news—emotionally and physically. Your body has enough to do without dealing with alien bags of chemicals shoved into it. Your mind has better things to occupy it than self-loathing and fear of what might go wrong. If somebody else thinks your breasts are "too small," I think we know who's really got the problem. After all, what self-respecting gal would trash her bosom buddies?

◉

Collagen implants Collagen, fat from cows collected in the blood and din of an abattoir, is injected under the skin, usually to make a fat lip, also known as Paris Lip, or Oh My God Have You Run Into A Door Handle? It costs about $300 to $500 and can also be injected into wrinkles to plump them out.

A test patch is always done first to check for any allergy. Usually the collagen is injected into the arm, and they'll charge you from $50 to $75 for that. If there is no reaction after a month, the service is performed.

The effect is temporary. The body absorbs all the collagen within two to six months. In April 1992, a magazine reported that the Food and Drug Administration made collagen manufacturers put a warning on their product that customers who have autoimmune disorders should not use it. Collagen manufacturers maintain that cow collagen cannot cause the human immune system to attack itself, so it cannot start an autoimmune problem. There is no long-term study on the effects of animal collagen used in this way.

The surgeons Sydney cosmetic surgeon Dr. Darryl Hodgkinson told a magazine that he was initially sceptical about laser surgery. The first lasers, he said, were "massive and not that easy to control. Also, they heated the surrounding skin up so much there was a lot of charred tissue."

Another thing Dr. Hodgkinson didn't like was the fact that customers—people —bruised. "One of the problems in our work is morbidity, the swelling and bruising patients experience after surgery. We do everything we possibly can—select patients carefully, get them off aspirin, talk to them about proper nutrition, 'ice' them on the table—but they still bruise." He became convinced that laser surgery could reduce bruising.

But the body will bruise if you hurt it. That's what it's for, it's the body's way of recovering after an injury. It's an injury that plastic surgeons might call "treatment." In the United States, lasers can be used by doctors untrained in their use. This apparent danger to customers is opposed by the American Society of Plastic and Reconstructive Surgeons. Dr. Leo Rozner, a member of the Australian Society of Plastic Surgeons, likens his practice to virtual reality. He says, "The technology is available and the pressures of fashion and compliance influence people. They can see the ideal face any day on television. It's rubbish that surgeons use their patients. The patients ask for what they want and they must be fully informed and research the matter. We are fixing deformities. Surgeons won't touch on schizoids or dysmorphics [people who are obsessed with tiny parts of themselves]." But *Webster's Collegiate Dictionary* defines "deform" as what Dr. Rozner is paid to do: "to spoil the form of; to spoil the looks of; disfigure."

On the subject of breasts, "Boobs go in and out of fashion but I have had a suit for 20 years and it has been in fashion three times. It depends what's happening but it can give women confidence and acceptability. Some are happy with the porky look."

He is unhappy with the media image of plastic surgeons. "We are reputable. We don't do anything without informed consent. The demands and the technology are growing in leaps and bounds. Melbourne has had its share of disasters [he named a cosmetic surgeon who killed a few customers with botched liposuction] but the technology is like a Mercedes. You don't get a 12-year-old to drive it."

He advises customers to look at the doctor's track record (I suppose you could knock on the door of his previous customers and demand to see their nipples) and build up a rapport with the doctor in time, before deciding. "There are risks of course. You buy a car and there are no guarantees that you won't have an accident. Never do business with a person you don't like, whether it's second-hand cars or second-hand faces," he says.

I do not suggest that all plastic surgeons are disreputable or sneaky or that they cajole customers into unwanted operations, although I am quite sure these things have happened. I do suggest that somebody who talks about the "porky" look, who compares women's bodies to suits and cars, and medical procedures to a Mercedes, is not a person I care to agree with. I found Dr. Rozner to be honest, helpful, and charming. But he too believes that women are "deformed" by the natural process of ageing, or if they have small breasts. I think that sucks.

In his *Avenue Cosmetic Plastic Surgery Health Update* newsletter to customers, Dr. Rozner describes a person's cosmetic surgery as a job prerequisite. "It is now part of the investment in their work, rather like dressing up for the office. It is also an investment in themselves as their prestige and success in employment are important and closely linked with their looks. You never, ever get a second chance to make a good impression at a job interview."

His brochure offers, "If desired, Asian features can be softened by enlarging the nose and making it narrower, by reducing the flare of the nostrils and by lifting the bridge of the nose to make it a more prominent feature. A double eyelid can be achieved by reducing skin and fat to make the fold higher," and "we aim for excellence and occasionally achieve perfection." One can only hope that Asian girls and women don't take this seriously.

Dr. Rozner says surgery can improve a person's image, and seems completely unaware of the chilling nature of his statement, "In many instances, facial cosmetic surgery is psychiatry with a knife."

chapter four

Fashion victims

Models and role models

Heroines Books and magazines for girls have always been full of role models: some interesting, some screamingly tedious. Girls' annuals from England, a staple reading diet for Australian girls until about the 1960s, were always full of daring schoolgirls catching smugglers or solving crimes, or exploring vast, "unexplored" wildernesses otherwise quite familiar to the indigenous people, or slaughtering another team at hockey. Nancy Drew, the schoolgirl detective in Carolyn Keene's novels, was also an adventurer.

Not that I'm suggesting that we should all go back to reading Nancy Drew books, but at least there were some roles for women. They actually *did* things. They didn't just stand around looking at the camera trying to sell you an A-line frock. Now our role models are more likely to be presented as simply silent, involved in nothing more challenging than pouting, or riding a bike, as long as it's just to tone up the thighs and not necessarily to go anywhere. Books for teenage girls are often just about how to find a guy (or how to lose one and get another). Models may be smart, funny women, but that's not why they're famous.

We have to find our own role models by discovering books

with real heroines, movies about feisty women, stories of girls and women who do more than drape themselves over half a palm tree in a $200 bikini.

Magazines point out the different definitions of beauty we have for actresses and models. They have freckles and gaps in their teeth and they range from brunettes to blondes, with short hair or long. We are told that there is far more individuality now than there used to be. But look at what all those varied faces do have in common. Overwhelmingly they're white and, even more overwhelmingly, they are all carried by thin bodies. They don't reflect all of us. It is the same for TV stars, for newsreaders, for almost any woman allowed onto our screens.

Actress Andie MacDowell says, "They only want you if you have a voice like a woman, a body like a girl and a mind like a man... If one more person asks me to lose five pounds, I'm going to be sick. I don't want to go through it any more and I don't want my daughter to go through it either. We've made some progress, but not much."

The images of women and girls that we see on television are completely censored. Any woman photographed for a magazine is photographed with a lot of makeup, usually a photographer with instructions to flatter her, and, in the case of American magazines, often a retouch job as well. Very often, famous people have a power of veto over which photographs of themselves are used. Authors usually choose their own publicity photographs (I personally destroyed the one of me wearing only an undershirt on the bunny rug).

The associate photo editor of a famous celebrity magazine in New York won't give celebrities power of veto but she will ask them what they're worried about and look out for it herself, including "lines on their neck or whatever." The editor, who wants to remain anonymous, says most things are taken care of in the *two hours* usually allotted for hair and makeup before the photography begins. She feels that retouching a photograph if a chin looks weird because of the way the light hits it is no different from setting up lights in the first place. "It's just another phase in the whole thing, and it's not real. None of it is real."

She can remember the time a famous rock star had her armpits made up and she trusted her personal makeup artist so much she didn't bother looking in the mirror when he was finished. "He

> The boys at my school are just waiting for the next Elle Macpherson to walk through the door. One guy even collects Elle memorabilia and had a scrapbook with her pictures in it. The boys are 14 to 15-ish and very immature. They will wake up when they realise the shortage of Elles in this world. Why can't we have healthy role models of all sizes, so it's fair to everyone? Why does everyone have this Beauty Thing? It is like a curse and eventually wrecks people's lives.
>
> Kelly, 14

was completely transforming her face...accentuating the eyes, the cheekbones and all that stuff but to a much greater degree, which looks kind of weird in person, but on film it works." And the cost? " Probably the more run-of-the-mill portrait without too much of an entourage is $1500, $2000, depending on how much everybody charges. The photographers make the most money.

"One of the things I find interesting is how you have this really long time to do hair and makeup and there doesn't look like there is any on, you know there's a *lot* of makeup but it's so...it's an illusion. All it's done has changed something, but you can't put your finger on it. It's a painting, it's truly a painting at that point. One makeup guy works with many divas: he paints. It's not like you or I would put lipstick on.

"The other thing that's interesting is when you go ohhh, they've really messed them up, they 've got so much makeup on they look like shit and then in the photographs it doesn't look like that, it just looks like they 're beautiful...you don't put makeup on men, you might put a little bit, but mostly what you do with a guy is you'll just put a bit of powder on them so there is no shine in the lights. And then the hair gets done." Later, changes may be made to the photographs on a computer screen.

> TV and magazines: to me, I see all those gorgeous models and I think, "Wow. She's got a great bod! I wish!"
>
> Sal, 19

Coathangers These days, the beauty-contest replacement seems to be cover -girl contests where young girls aspire to be models or disembodied, disembrained "faces of the year." These contests are often sponsored by modelling agencies who help choose the winner and then start making money out of her. Being a model is almost always presented as something glamorous and exciting and wonderful.

Only about 5 to 10 percent of women are in the height and weight range of models. Most models are around 5'9" tall and wear a size 6 or 8 dress, and have a bust size of 33 to 34 inches, bra cup A or B, waist 25 to 26 inches, and hips 35 to 36. Models must also have unusually wide shoulders. Cindy Crawford is almost 29 pounds lighter than the average woman of her height: 5'9" and size 6. "I think women see me on the cover of magazines and think I never have a pimple or bags under my eyes," says Ms. Crawford. "You have to realise that's after two hours of hair and makeup, plus [photo] retouching. Even *I* don't wake up looking like Cindy Crawford."

A reporter at the New York fashion collections looks at the women on the catwalks and concludes, "There are no thighs in sight—it's hard to believe these women are the same species as me, let alone the same gender."

Somewhere along the line, the thin girls who had shoulders like coathangers became not just models but "supermodels" and, even more puzzling, role models. They are asked for beauty hints, opinions, and space-filling quotes. None of this is memorable unless it is arrogant ("We don't get out of bed for less than $10,000 a day," said Linda Evangelista) or stupid (asked why there are no books in her apartment, Elle Macpherson said, "I don't think you should read what you haven't written"). None of it is important because of what is being said, only because of who is saying it.

This year's models Almost all models are told what to wear, what to do with their hair, how to look, how to act, what kind of an image to project—in short, what kind of a person they are. Models are "managed," treated like children, possibly because some of them are. Models are, excuse the language, treated like shit.

The truth is, models *are* some of the most insecure, tortured souls around. The industry likes them that way. They're more likely to always do what they're told: look blank or perky. Perkily blank, maybe. Or blankly perky. That's about the range.

Many models *are* smart. It's just that their job does not reward them for it.

At an American model convention, one agent wants 15-year-old skin for cosmetics ads while another addresses girls waiting in line to see him. He likes only "one or two. One and a half. The second half I have to talk to my plastic surgeon." The girl, 15, will be told by a modelling agency in her hometown that she has no future unless she has an operation on her nose.

Model Lynn Snowden told *Esquire* magazine, "Models have such an obsession with minor flaws. The average receptionist has a better self-image than the average model." A modelling agent explains how he treats the women who keep him in business. "Never, ever compliment them. They're complimented constantly by losers. It's sick, but this is an inside thing. If you mention something that's an imperfection about them, say, a mole, or their hair looks bleached—they're yours." Another top agent told *New York* magazine that when girls get older they start to think for themselves too much.

Models are never called women; only girls, no matter how old or how smart they are.

It must be easy to get things out of proportion when eating anything at all is seen as some kind of weakness. Teenage model Tanya Arpadi told a magazine that she loves food and doesn't worry about her weight. Yet she describes having a cup of tea and some toast after school as "pigging out." Her only other reference to eating, in front of the telly, is also described as "pigging out." It is as if any consumption of food at all is presented as greed.

Lingerie modelling can be very high paying, which may motivate many models to get breast implants. Inevitably, the models themselves, as individuals, cop it from the press, even from a magazine which once idolised them. "The pumped up hair and breasts and stature of [the 1980s supermodels] symbolises the excesses of the 1980s," said *Allure*. Australian *Cleo* called the waifs "snotty stringbeans in their skimpy, wimpy threads."

> I open a magazine and a supermodel stares back at me, her waist the size of a Life Saver. An article accompanying the picture constantly mentions how beautiful she is. I immediately drop the magazine and start doing sit-ups. Can you blame me?
>
> Sarah

Magazines now run stories on models as they used to on movie stars. Australian *Dolly* has a regular tear-out double postcard of a male and female model in each issue. Obviously, the obsession with models is selling magazines. We learn from lists of their characteristics in Australian *Cosmopolitan* that "virtues" include "always keeps her skin looking perfect," "avoids partying," and "doesn't drink coffee." Vices include "chocolates and croissants," "ice-cream," "junk food," "a tendency to flirt," and "sweet foods." Eating and flirting! Vices! Give me a break!

The makeup job on models "*Harper's Bazaar* retouches photographs of girls like crazy. Other magazines too. They just take out any imperfections. They'll slim a girl's hips or lengthen her legs. They can do anything now," a New York makeup artist says. "When you're doing their makeup you can see...like they're really heavy under the eyes, really dark, and the girls who have lines around their eyes—and you see the picture [in the magazine] and it's completely smooth, or maybe their eyes were bloodshot that day, the eyes are real bright and white. It's amazing what you can do even [with makeup]."

waifer - thin

The endless cycle The first fashion parade models, in London in 1900, were all tall and big. None of them weighed less than 155 pounds, and "several of them considerably more."

Lately models are tall and thin. Big breasts are sometimes "fashionable," sometimes not.

In the 1960s the first waifs were personified by Englishwomen Penelope Tree and Twiggy (Lesley Hornby). In the early 1990s they were Kate Moss and Australian Emma Balfour. Kate Moss, at 106 pounds and 5'7" tall, is unusually short for modelling and underweight by all health and medical guidelines. But she has coathanger shoulders. Magazine editors called the waifs the "cut-price models," those who work for thousands of dollars less than their predecessors in their eagerness to become as well known.

Emma Balfour says she sometimes worries about the effect waif-worship has on young girls. "When I feel fat I don't eat so much," this very skinny girl told a magazine interviewer.

> I also feel pressure from magazines. They advertise clothes for people maybe 15 and up, but they use these 12, 13-year-old models who haven't even started puberty yet. How are we supposed to compete with girls who have boys' bodies?
>
> Melissa, 15

Those in the industry seem to want to have it both ways: the bigger models make women feel better about themselves, but the waifs have no effect at all. Richard Harper, director of Cameron's actors and models agency in Sydney, says he is violently against the waif look. Elle Macpherson, he said, "served as a catalyst. Suddenly girls could have a shape." Later in the same interview he said women do not change to suit fashion. "I don't take responsibility for any of it and what's more I've never yet met a woman who'd do anything I wanted her to do."

Harper's Bazaar ran a seven-page feature claiming that the waifs were so thin only because of genes and "hard work." Penelope Tree says she was a miserable anorexic at the height of her period of fame and adulation as a 1960s waif model. In some photographs of her at the time, she looks remarkably like Kate Moss, the same hollow cheeks and dull eyes—and indeed designer Calvin Klein says he first booked Moss because she reminded him of Penelope Tree, more "real" than the bigger supermodels.

Harper's Bazaar defended its use of the waif models against outraged letters from readers. "What you're seeing on our pages is not a horde of starvation-riven women. This is an ectomorphic body type. It's in fashion... Eating disorders are not new complaints. People were dieting long before newsstands were invented."

Cleo was horrified and called it "the fashion look that should carry a health warning... They might be in, but at what cost?...The blank-slate waifs of the 1990s, with their empty, childlike attitude, are helplessness personified. The look may be 1970s grunge, but the message is pure 1950s helplessness."

Allure magazine cited the waifs as "the triumph of poverty, of vulnerability." Kate Moss's photographer Corinne Day said, "I love reality—things like bad posture, vacant stares, skinniness." (Drug addiction, war, famine, tennis anybody?) Dress designer Valentino said, "I love these young, new girls, frail and insecure." (Creep.) *Harper's Bazaar* concluded, "Like to be Kate Moss? We all would." Speak for yourself.

Modelling agent Eileen Ford sneers at the very idea that the idealisation of models might have a bad influence. "Models do not have a negative impact on women. They have a positive impact because they set standards. Women are going to look like themselves but they will look like their best selves because models set standards. When you think you look your best, and feel your best, there's an aura around you of self-confidence and self-assurance. Models do that to women." What models did to one reporter at the New York fashion shows in 1993, she said, was make her feel "fat and malformed all week."

> I try to like myself for what I am but I open up a magazine and immediately compare myself with those perfect models.
>
> Jacquiline, 17

It was reported that the bigger models were dieting to be even thinner, to compete. The thinner models make the others feel scared. A New York makeup artist told me of working on a shoot with a well-known model. "The day I worked with her, all day long she was hungry, so hungry. I said, well, eat something, do you want me to get you a bagel or something? 'No, no, no, I can't eat, I can't eat, I can't eat. I can't work if I eat.' And that was just crazy. She finally had a sip of orange juice at four o'clock. She's so thin, so thin...I think a lot of them do drugs because I don't think there's any way you can be that thin without doing something. I have seen lots of photographs of [a famous model] when she had got really anorexic but a lot of the time they are dressed and you don't really see it. Her waist was the size of my thigh, probably thinner."

The makeup artist said she sometimes has to camouflage the skin of a waif. "I tend to give them colour so they look more alive. Sort of like a heroin addict...when you are that thin it's hard to keep your skin good, you need lots of aids."

Diane Parks, the Australian editor of *Slimming* magazine, says: "[F ashion photography] is like food photography, you tart it up a bit because you don't have the other things that go with real food, like taste and smell. With pictures of models, you don't get those other parts about meeting human beings, like personality."

> Whenever I open magazines I look at the models. They are so lucky to have a perfect body and perfect skin. Like the girls in the pictures advertising L'Oréal products. I recently had this guy kissing me and all that stuff that happens and haven't heard from him since. It totally sucks.
>
> Lottie, 14

Tortured models Models rarely admit to having eating disorders until their modelling careers are over. Australian *Who Weekly* magazine ran a cover story called "The Price of Beauty," a story of "supermodels" Carol Alt, Beverly Johnson, and Kim Alexis, in which the three women detailed their low self -esteem, "nightmare diets," and "vicious treatment on the job." Success meant "a constant gnawing hunger ." "They met the enemy and it was food." The healthy image was attained with lighting, makeup, and a public brainwashed to believe that thin was always healthy .

Kim Alexis said the head of the Elite Modelling agency "guaranteed me a certain amount of money if I lost 15 pounds." Carol Alt was a straight-A student when a photographer noticed her . The first agent she contacted "told me I'd be perfect if I lost 15 pounds."

Ms. Alexis says, "I remember trying every fad diet. I remember starving myself for four days in a row ." She shared a flat with model Kelly Emberg. "One night I was eating only a head of lettuce for dinner. Kelly walked in and said, 'You're eating a *whole* head of lettuce? How could you?' I cried and said 'But it's all I've had all day. It's not even 50 calories.'

"I think I was a normal person before I started screwing around with these diets. My metabolism got screwed up. I lost my period for two full years...I'd dread lunch [during a shoot] because the client would look at me and say , 'You're not going to eat that are you?" Carol Alt says, "Do you remember the Beverly Hills diet? You only ate fruit. It was terrible. A t another point I was drinking eight cups of coffee a day and I ate salad for dinner. On my first modelling job I fainted. An editor had given me one month to lose 11 pounds. If I did she promised me a trip to Rome... So I stopped eating. Maybe I'd have celery, an apple. I went along doing the one salad a night routine for a year. I remember feeling so tired and depressed. I had no personal life...eventually I learned to eat five small meals a day."

"In our profession clothes look better on a hanger, so you have to look like a clothes hanger. It will never change," said Beverly Johnson.

147

Why don't they show bigger models?

It seems that magazines only use size-8 models because the designers and manufacturers only give them size-8 samples to photograph. The magazine editors do not challenge this, and a stereotype is maintained.

But the real reason why models are size 8 has nothing to do with what is acceptable in real life and *everything* to do with all the money to be made by the fashion industry, which still calls the shots, provides the samples, and creates an atmosphere of envy to help sell their product.

Carlotta Moye, fashion editor of *Dolly* magazine says, "We are working a season ahead and there is only one sample... We had a 15-year-old on a photo shoot and she put on seven pounds on the trip and the pictures just did not look good—she put it on in the boobs and hips and she lost her aspirational appeal. We had to crop the picture below the waist... She has lost it now and she's back to her perfect self...she only just got her period a few months ago.

"There isn't just one body shape in the magazines—things change. I don't go for weight when I choose models, I go for personality. Weight ranks maybe third or fourth on the list of requirements. Sometimes we get letters saying models look too skinny. Some people say we should make her look fatter. Women are very critical and bitchy. They never criticise hair colour but they are obsessed with weight."

According to *Vogue* Australian fashion editor Victoria Collison, "Clothes look better on those small-size girls. You are presenting a look, an image... Clothes can look good on most sized models though. Every May–June we do a working women's story, the strong career women with clothes to fit them—larger than size six or eight—it is a more realistic image, and this is the way we can cover it. The size eight thing has always happened that way. These clothes could look just as good on a size 12 if she is tall. A magazine has a certain amount of fantasy."

Girlfriend fashion editor Catherine Murphy says, "We try to avoid the skinny look if we can because we are aware of the anorexia issue but I think the illness itself is more complex than just the image thing. With fashion there is a lot of choice now, girls are wearing more boys' clothes. We usually do two stories with bigger and smaller girls. Our readers are younger and slightly smaller anyway. Obviously models are thin and personally I feel strongly about the anorexia issue. Society wants to see then this way [size 8]—that is what the girls want; [size] 12 to 14 is not what they perceive as attractive. Designers see that their garments look better on proportionally thin, taller models."

> I don't know whether I should stay with the muscly toned look or the waif look. Sometimes I wish supermodels didn't exist and body shape didn't matter because then you wouldn't have to keep up. Since I got weighed in P.E. class everyone, including the teacher, thinks I'm extremely underweight and no one wants to help me with a diet. Why doesn't someone help me with a healthy diet that will help me lose weight and make me look like one of those models? Because I know I'd feel better about myself if I did.
>
> Anonymous
>
> My boyfriend has supermodels all over his walls, which is a little annoying, but he always reassures me.
>
> Lena, 19

"Aspirational appeal"—the atmosphere of envy—seems to be the key here. Fashion editors are choosing what they think we want to be. While the designers are the only ones who will provide the sample clothes and buy the fashion ads in magazines, nothing much will change unless magazine readers *en masse* demand a change. Unsurprisingly perhaps, given their jobs, most fashion editors do not question the notion that different body shapes can be "in fashion" while the shape of real people stays pretty much the same for each individual.

So, if we want bigger models in the magazines, we have to write and tell them. "Dear Editor, the model on page 72 of your latest issue looks like a sick whippet. I want to know what the clothes will look like on a size 14. And PS, please give that model some lunch before she faints. Signed, Reasonably Outraged Come to Think About It."

The fashion industry

Girly lures Stores such as The Limited, Strawberry, and Express have been made into one-stop girly lures, offering everything under the one roof: shoes, undies, accessories, hairclips, jewellery. Each store tries to create an image, a readymade made-up lifestyle. In some it is pop music interspersed with ads for their products and blow-up photographs of models, often with accessories, including a boyfriend (*not* in stock). The shops provide casual clothes, going-out clothes, and, sometimes, work clothes. Shops such as The Limited suggest a mix-and-match wardrobe, especially for work.

Then there are the designer shops with higher price tags and often better cuts, fabrics, and more carefully finished clothes. But not always. Women are encouraged by advertising and image-making to choose a designer or two and stick with them: to have a look created for them, rather than finding clothes that go with their look, their per - sonality, and their activities.

It is relatively easy to track general fashion. Fashion is usually worn by the young: people in their teens and early twenties who have the money to change their wardrobe and are more likely to be bothered by what others think of them. Style is different altogether: a personal style that suits the personality and pursuits of the wearer and is not dictated by anybody else.

In 1994 total retail sales for the American fashion and footwear industries were estimated at $246.5 billion. The number of people employed is falling constantly, due to the government policies that allow unrestricted importing of clothes from overseas, which is cheaper because the people making them are paid about a nickel and a sardine a month.

> You always see in movies a perfect guy and a beautiful woman making out anywhere they please. They aren't at all realistic, the women always have beautiful clothes, not just shorts and a T-shirt: matching undies and bras, not the cheap ones where the elastic or wire is falling out!
>
> Tina, 16

According to one television series about the fashion industry, it's a $975 billion a year industry worldwide.

So the clothes stores are competing with each other to get you to buy their clothes. They will do this by telling you through their ads and magazines that you *need* their clothes.

The boom boom Lately (not that you wouldn't have noticed, dear, pass the turnip) we have been having a recession. F or instance, bra sales fell by $9 million in 1987, just when we were being told there was a huge boom in lingerie. Mind you, we are told every year that there's a boom in lingerie. My definition of a boom is not a $9 million drop in sales, but this is possibly the reason I am not in marketing. There seems to be only a boom in booms, if you know what I mean.

Fashion manufacturers create the styles and then try to convince us to buy them. This is why everything changes so dramatically from one season to the next—bright neon colours one summer, sandy, mushroomy colours the next, so one bit won't match the rest the next time you buy something.

One way manufacturers try and boost sales is the self-proclaimed boom, that staple tactic of the lingerie industry promoters. They've been doing it since at least 1952 when National Corset Week was announced. Recently a manufacturer claimed that women were rushing to buy inflatable bras with a little attachment like a bike pump. Oh, say it ain't so!

For a few years now, spurred on by Madonna's conical, comical boobs jutting out from a designer corset, manufacturers have been trying to sell us thousands of "bustiers": a new-fashioned corset, only slightly more comfy than the whalebone-and-rubber monstrosities of the past that had women fainting, in floods of sweat and with internal damage. When *Allure* magazine did a fashion spread on them, even the fashion writer had to admit, "It took six hands, all pulling in different directions, to fit the actress [*actress!!?*] photographed here in three bustiers by Valentino. And the largest waist was an enviable 25 inches," she wrote, betraying only her own envy. She continued, "there is probably nothing more beautiful than the contours of bare shoulders and barely concealed breasts." That woman should take a holiday somewhere where you can get scenery.

The Lee jeans company responded cleverly to the piffle about bustiers with a series of ads aimed at real women. "Corsets. Girdles. High heels. Isn't it time women's clothes were designed for women?" the ad headline implored. The copy continued, "How could any sane woman, for example, no matter how proud of her torso, have possibly dreamed up the bustier? What about the girdle [named after the sound you make when you try to put one on]...since women come in different shapes, there are several fits of...jeans available to women...[including] relaxed fit jeans and loose fit. Try finding a relaxed fit corset."

> Jennifer: "So today I'm joined by Dawn French, top fashion expert to the stars and the high street. So tell me, Dawn, what can we expect to see in the shops this year?"
>
> Dawn: "Clothes mostly...and some hats and some shoes."
>
> Comedians Jennifer Saunders and Dawn French

It is said that Marie Antoinette invented the idea of pushing her bosoms up somewhere around her chin in a low-cut frock, and she certainly didn't have much else to do. Ungaro, a designer, "invented" a body suit which exposed all of the back, and (I'm about to be indelicate, turn the page if you are easily shocked, thank you) what is politely known as the buttock cleft, otherwise as the butt crack.

Designers who show bosom-twisting cleavage and butt-exposing jumpsuits cannot seriously expect us to wear these things.

The publicity game What they are doing is getting the pictures of their models in the fashion magazines and on television. The more shocking and, whoopsie there's a nipple, outrageous the better. Almost any publicity is good publicity. Perhaps only two copies of that ridiculous dress exist but many more copies of the photo do.

There, in the magazine, a pouting 15-year-old, with a long slash of dark purple on each eyebrow, is wearing an open hospital gown, with an old garbage bag held together with a bulldog clip wrapped around her chest. She is wearing a pair of shorts made from muslin stapled to an old wheat sack. Nobody will ever wear it again. The model certainly wouldn't be seen dead in it unless she was getting paid $2,500 for the day.

But the designer has made a splash in an industry where there must be something new every minute. The designer's other collection, called "ready to wear," will indeed be more "wearable" and copied by factory owners in Southeast Asia. We'll get a watered-down version of it by spring, and an ad with a picture of a happy young girl wearing it, who is oblivious to the clothes and with her arm around a *boyfriend* (pause for round of applause).

When there are see-through clothes for the office on the catwalk, and the designers suggest long, tight skirts with scarily high heels for women who have to use public transport to get home, we know most people won't really buy them. Manufacturers have tried several times since the 1960s to bring back the "baby doll" dress for grown-ups and adolescents: it is very rarely seen except in advertisements and on the pages of magazines. Oh, and on baby dolls.

ZELDA DEMONSTRATES THE ACCEPTABLE TECHNIQUE FOR STEPPING OUT OF PLATFORM-SOLED SHOES. (DEGREE of DIFFICULTY; 8·9)

Scary shoes If you must wear high heels, don't wear them every day. They are a known cause or encourager of hammer toes, bunions, corns, and lower leg and back problems. Most women don't develop these foot and related problems until their late teens when they start wearing high heels. High heels put two and a half times more weight onto some of the bones in the foot than if you were barefoot. Constant wearing of high heels causes the Achilles tendon to shrink, and then when you switch to smaller heels or sport shoes, it can be very painful. Platform shoes are completely stupid.

Further reading

Nicholas Coleridge, *The Fashion Conspiracy: A Remarkable Journey through the Empires of Fashion* (New York: Harper & Row, 1988). A fabulously entertaining and well-written book which exposes how the whole thing really works.

Lyn Schnurnberger, *Let There Be Clothes* (New York: Workman, 1991). A history of fashion. Not too much text, lots of illustrations and explanations of where what came from.

Style police

Domina-tricks The style police don't even have a uniform we can recognise them by. (This is only one of the infuriating things about them.) They might be wearing some frightfully expensive tweedy togs with batwing sleeves or a wee bit of cheesecloth draped about their private parts, but they have one thing in common: they think they are the boss of us.

The style police tell us what we should wear—as a matter of fact, what we *must* wear and also what we are not allowed to wear. I'll be the first to admit there are clothes I think should be dropped off in a bottomless quarry on Saturn. But there *are* people who like to wear lime green stretch polyester and orange A-line frocks, and good luck to them.

The style police think that what we look like is more important than anything (*particularly* world peace) and it is their job to seek out and punish those who break their own fashion rules. Some of them are obviously stupid: "I consider that without hats, an intrinsic part of fashion, we would have no civilisation," said dressmaker and numbskull Christian Dior in 1957.

And therein lies a clue to why the style police behave in such a way. There are many different squads in the style police. There are designers, sellers, and advertisers of clothes who will make money out of selling an "essential" item or style. Another style cop is the catty person who wants to feel herself the most stylish person

INTRODUCING: SOCIAL **BLUNDER WOMAN**

Last night, on a date, she laughed with her mouth full and café latte came out of her nose.

socks with sandals

KAZ

around. If she knocks your style she can feel better about her own. There are also fashion writers and freelance journalists filling up space around the ads in magazines and newspapers.

Come with me into the bossy-boots world of the style police. Carry a stout stick and don't be afraid to lay about yourself with it if you see any battalions of fashion writers whining about how our clothes look at least 17 minutes out of date. Come with me first into one of the most obvious areas of the style police: the wedding organisers. No! No! Oh, all right, I promise we won't be here long.

Oh my *Lord*: have you ever seen so many rules in all your *life*? The dress has to be white. The dress has to be cream. The dress has to be elegant and simple. The dress has to be feminine and frilly. The dress has to look like a dangerous explosion in an organza factory during a cyclone. There must be expensive flowers. There must be an expensive photographer. You must have your facial three days before the wedding, your hair done, your nails done, your makeup done, blah, blah, and quite frankly, more blah. (And have you read our sensational *Blah Supplement?*)

The wedding dress is usually at the end of each haute couture show, the most expensive item, the climax of the show, as in days gone past, and in some quarters, a wedding is supposed to be the climax of a lifetime.

Take a closer look at that special supplement about the right way to get married. Look at all those advertisements around it and scattered through it. What a con. If you want to carry roses from your Aunty Levitatia's garden and get married in a nice old dress you found at the thrift shop, you do it. The only ones screaming will be those you might have hired or bought from if you'd swallowed the "rules," which were mostly made up by people who profit from them.

Fashion crime and fashion criminals In the space-filling, get-somebody-else-to-do-most-of-the-thinking-for-this-article tradition of journalism (hey, I know about this, I've done it myself) comes the "50 all-time fashion disasters according to the experts" type of story, and of course the snide "worst dressed" lists and photographs with nasty captions in women's magazines. This kind of stuff makes us all into the style police. We can say, hey, that actor may have millions of dollars but she looks absolutely shocking in a puce velvet Heidi frock. It's the revenge of the ordinary against the (literally) well-heeled.

The opposite to this is the designers and clothes sellers telling us what's a fashion "crime." This is the revenge of the well-heeled on the ordinary—a chance for fashion designers to get really annoyed at us for not doing everything they tell us.

One newspaper, prompted by its panel of experts (almost all of them clothes manufacturers and sellers), says we can't wear body-hugging dresses if we "don't have the right body to hug." The wrong body, said the newspaper, has a "protruding bottom and tummy." Well, I do beg your pardon, but if your bottom

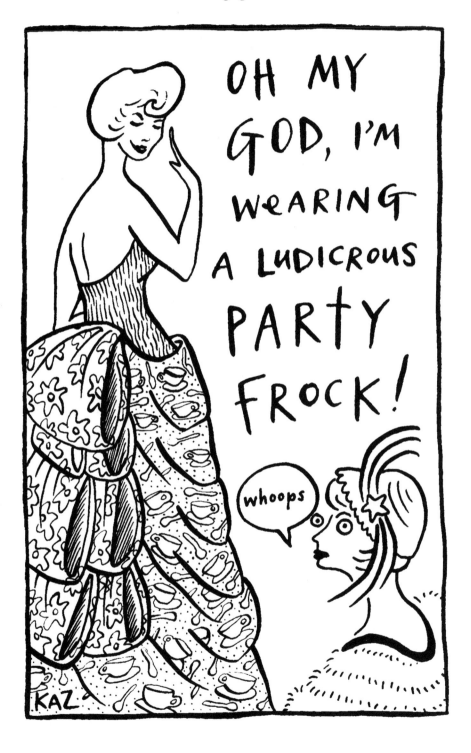

doesn't protrude you've probably lost it entirely, in which case I suggest you contact a doctor .

Of course, this sort of thing is passed off as helpful hints, like the "right" swimsuit to wear to "camouflage" the body's "defects." Or, as one magazine more kindly put it, "to show off your good points." Various drawings of women are shown with the "right" and the "wrong" swimsuit for each to wear. For example, the "wrong" swimsuit for the "pear-shaped" woman (that is, most adult women) has horizontal stripes.

The "right" one apparently has a kind of a scarfy arrangement at the top, draped over the shoulders and tied between the breasts and three different colours on the rest of it with a stripe pointing down like an arrow at about waist level and a dark section below the waist. A swimsuit even vaguely resembling this has never been seen by me on any swimsuit racks. And I have been through a lot of them, looking for something plain and black that does not have leg holes cut up to just underneath the armpits.

Fashion writers From a consumer's point of view, a good fashion writer will present new clothes, classics, and a range of what's available at a range of prices, using photographs that show the clothes accurately on people who are shaped like the consumers. But from an advertiser's point of view, a good fashion writer runs glamorous pictures of its clothes and makes them look desirable and different. This is often done by photographing them in front of some children in a "travel" location, which keeps the tourism industry advertisers and the photo crew (including the fashion writer) happy as well.

We should be very careful of who is telling us what to wear on our bodies and on our faces. As photographer Bruce Weber says of the three writers he admires the most, "What these women really have in common is that they're styling what their life is, what *their own* lives are about." It's very scary when these women

—An English fashion designer told me to wear high heels with jeans. Should I listen?

—No.

Writer Cynthia Heimel

just might be insecure, neurotic, unhappy, too busy to consider the rights and wrongs of what they are doing and are subject to the whims of advertisers in their magazines.

A high-powered international fashion editor goes to the collections and private showings. She chooses some clothes.

She organises a contra-deal, that is, a free trip to somewhere exotic in return for free "plugs" for the tourist resort in the magazine. Once there, she unpacks the clothes, the models, hopes the photographer won't get malaria, and gaffer-tapes the backs of the frocks to make them sit just right on the thin models. She tries to make the shoot "interesting," perhaps even "creative," or chooses a photographer with such ambitions.

Sometimes she tells you in the text next to the photo that something's an "essential." This could be a white shirt, a ruched tulle skirt with velour tassels, or a hairpin with a plastic daisy on it. Sometimes the fashion editor is desperate. But the fashion editor is never, ever, infallible. Sometimes she says stupid things about stupid clothes and changes her mind by autumn.

> Keep a pair of high-heeled slippers in your bathroom.
>
> Britt Ekland
>
> Keep a porcupine in your underpants—it would be more comfortable.
>
> Hermoine the Modern Girl

That's her job.

I was a fashion writer at a newspaper for about three weeks. If it ever happens to you and you don't want to be a fashion editor, here's what you do. Run a story with pictures of a Paris designer's coat (about $1,200) and the local department store's coat (about $500) and how you can make one yourself (about $70), and wait for the Paris designer's shop and the department store, a big advertiser in your newspaper, to throw a mega-fit. You will not be a fashion editor for long.

Vogue magazine is regarded as an arbiter of fashion. At last count it was charging more than $50,000 for a full-page advertisement and was making more than $112 million a year. That's 112 million reasons not to upset the advertisers.

Longtime icon and *Vogue* editor Diana Vreeland once (although she was at *Harper's Bazaar* at the time) decided to write a new fashion law. "We're going to eliminate all handbags," she announced, explaining that designers would have to provide pockets in their clothes for women. At the time, this was pretty revolutionary. Someone was summoned to Vreeland to explain how things really worked. "I think you've lost your mind," she said diplomatically. "Do you realise our income from handbag advertising is God knows how many millions a year?" Exactly. And *Harper's Bazaar* did not then announce the death of the handbag.

chapter five

Hyper hype

Lotions and potions

Big bucks First, we pause for a small mind boggle. American consumers spent almost $16 billion on cosmetics, toiletries, and perfumes in 1994.

Moisturisers and anti-wrinkle creams Skin specialists agree that a good moisturiser will temporarily smooth and "plump" out wrinkles only because it is adding water to the skin. This plumping-out effect makes no lasting change to skin, all of which, no matter what you slather on, is always getting older.

Asked whether expensive creams are better, they offer this cost-benefit analysis. "You might get a 90 percent improvement with [a generic] cream and a 95 percent improvement with something that costs 10 or 20 times as much." That 5 percent difference is probably not visible to the naked eye. Only 5 to 10 percent of people have a naturally dry skin and really "need" a moisturiser.

In 1986 the Australian Consumers' Association had 800 people use 90 over-the-counter moisturisers given to them in unlabelled bottles. A plain generic cream made from petrolatum, glycerine, and water, rated as high or higher than the expensive stuff with designer names.

When the "blind" test survey was repeated in 1991, the best

four included a Tania vitamin E cream from Australian Coles supermarkets at 63 cents per 3.5 ounces, Dermastine face cream with elastin at $60 per 3.5 ounces, Bio Swiss moisturiser from A ustralia at $16 per 3.5 ounces, and Herome skin conditioner from Holland at $45. The outright winner? The supermarket brand.

If you're a young woman, you probably won't care much about moisturisers until you're in your late twenties or early thir - ties. The simple truth is that a sunhat might save you thousands of dollars in creams and lotions. Especially if you don't drink heavily or smoke.

Dermatologists estimate that about 80 percent of what used to be thought normal ageing of the skin is actually "photo-ageing," due to exposure to sunlight. We are spending millions trying to correct it with creams and treatments that are scientifically un- able to repair the damage.

In America, most people over 45 have visible evidence of severe photo-ageing. You've probably seen the Luggage Women with skin like distressed leather and the Pink Men who look as if they get toasted every day.

This has to be balanced against sensible precautions and living a full life not locked away inside thinking what a nice skin you've got. But if you're actually baking in the sun, looking for a tan, you're looking for trouble.

What is a moisturiser? Moisturisers are either humectants, which add water to sit on top of the skin, or fats that form a "bar - rier" layer, making it harder for water in the skin to "evaporate" in air conditioning or in other drying environments. Either way, it's not particularly complicated. It's a case of "just add water "— you choose how much, which way, and the cost.

Dermatologists insist that the newer, extra ingredients in moisturisers, such as collagen and elastin, cannot be absorbed into the skin, despite the claims of cosmetic companies. Even Unilever's own chemist said collagen didn't do much of anything when rubbed into the top layer of skin. It's a molecule thing—like trying to get a yak through the hole in your mailbox.

Placentas—animal and, some say, human—were big for a while

as ingredients. Hyaluronic acid, introduced in the 1980s, is claimed to "deliver " more water to the skin. Then came "lipids" (just fats) and "liposomes," supposed to deliver ingredients below the upper surface of the epidermis (skin) but not necessarily do anything after they arrived (sort of like dull house guests).

Liposomes, teeny-weeny molecules, are the "taxis" used to deliver fancy ingredients below the surface of the skin. This allows moisturiser ads to use diagrams with arrows showing the moisturiser "getting into" the skin. But even liposome "taxis" will only take the moisturiser halfway. So far, no product can be delivered to the dermis, where the body makes its own collagen and elastin. And even if such a long-distance "taxi" were to be invented, there's no evidence that any added moisturiser at the dermis level would do anything except arrive.

Despite the fact that dermatologists and even the manufacturers of many cosmetics insist that, after billions of dollars of research over decades, not one— *not one*—potion has been invented that will interfere in any way with the ageing process, Australian *New Idea* magazine chose to run an article on cosmetic ingredients, headed "Anti-Ageing Breakthroughs."

The article gave the phone numbers of 13 cosmetics companies corresponding with the products mentioned. With friends like these you can reduce your advertising budget. But the magazine can't have been too sure about when to report a "breakthrough"—the article was published 18 months after it was written. The truth is that cosmetics companies announce "breakthroughs" on a regular basis as an advertising tool.

Buzzwords Ceramides A fat. Putting fat on the skin does not change the skin any more than peanut butter on a sandwich alters the state of the bread. *New Idea* still called ceramides "another breakthrough miracle ingredient."

Hyaluronic acid Made from roosters' combs. Dermatologists are sceptical of its ability to be absorbed properly once it is delivered to the epidermis. One likened the acid molecule to a length of piano wire and the skin to a bucket of water.

Liposomes These are fatty droplets extracted from eggs or from "plant extracts." But basically they're fat. One magazine called them "tiny, round, leakproof packages made of skin-friendly lipids." Oh, cute. Lipids are of course just fats. Dermatologists agree that liposomes only penetrate the upper skin. Some sellers of liposome products say that the product alters cells in the upper skin, but research from Christian Dior was not performed on human skin but on cells from mice spleens. (I don't know about you, but if there's one thing I can't stand it's a wrinkly mouse spleen.)

Elastin/collagen Normal skin at the dermis level contains elastin and collagen, which are damaged and altered by sunlight, possibly by UVB rays which are only stopped by opaque creams, clothing, or a solid hat. Added collagens and elastins usually come from animal fats and tissue. According to one Australian government health department spokesperson, "stuff like elastin has simply ginormous molecules. They simply can't get in."

Retin-A Retin-A (tretinoin cream based on retinoic acid, a vitamin A derivative) was developed as an acne cream, but was then sold in tens of millions of tubes over the counter as a new, amazing face-peeling wrinkle treatment. Other creams were also marketed with retinoic or tretinoic acid. More than one magazine called Retin-A a "miracle cream."

Many dermatologists said the cream improved the skin texture of test subjects and showed a reduction of wrinkles.

But Retin-A has also caused cancer in mice and an article in the English medical journal *The Lancet* told of three babies with birth defects—all the mothers had used vitamin A derivative therapeutic creams during pregnancy.

Retin-A damages the skin of some users, causing it to become red and inflamed and come off in flakes. This side effect "generally settles down" during or after use, according to the dermatologists. Another side effect is photosensitivity, so users should avoid the sun and use strong sunscreen.

The U.S. Food and Drug Administration has only approved Retin-A for acne treatment. In 1988, concerned by the enormous sales and overuse, the FDA commissioner issued a public warning about indiscriminate use of the drug for smoothing wrinkles. Since then, the company that makes Retin-A has produced a lower-strength formulation and done more tests in an attempt to get government approval to sell the drug as a wrinkle cream. An article in a medical journal in 1990 said: "Many dermatologists find that the topical treatment tretinoin (Retin-A) is their most frequently prescribed drug... However, it has not been approved by the FDA as an anti-wrinkle cream, although prescribing it for this purpose is considered 'accepted medical practice.'"

The makers of Retin-A say there is no link with cancer or birth defects. The company which distributes it in A ustralia sent a letter to pharmacists and doctors pointing to another *Lancet* article in May 1993 which showed that there was *not* a greater risk of defects in babies born to mothers who used Retin-A. The letter also pointed out that 45 million units of Retin-A had been sold in the United States in the last 20 years, and that the rate of deformities from unknown causes in the Australian community was 2 to 3 per - cent. The company concluded, "As with any drug, pregnant women should consult with their physicians before use, as the general recommendation is that Retin-A not be used in pregnancy or when pregnancy is likely."

Retin-A and its colleague products are, so far, the only truly "therapeutic" treatments available. "Therapeutic" doesn't mean it's necessarily good, it means that the product has been shown to change the body: in this case stimulating the generation of new collagen.

Acid trips Alpha hydroxy acids (AHAs) are found naturally in plants (often fruit) and dairy products. And now they're in cosmetics. They're another "miracle" being advertised. The acid is supposed to loosen the "glue" that binds dead cells to the skin's surface to reveal a fresher , new layer underneath.

When Estée Lauder launched a fruit-acid cream called Fruition, with much more extravagant claims than those made previously for fruit-acid products—"up to 18 percent reduction in the appearance of fine lines and wrinkles" and "60 percent increase in skin clarity "—it captured 10 percent of skin-care sales within weeks. Think about that 18 percent. Could you tell if a wrinkle looked 18 percent (about one-fifth) less deep?

Dermatologists point out that acid skin peels are done with very powerful acids that shouldn't be used unless under the care of a skin doctor. The glycolic acid used in a skin peel stings and burns when applied and is left for up to five minutes.

Even dermatologists admit that fruit acids cannot cure wrinkles, only diminish them in some cases over a period of time. And considering that wrinkles stay in the same place while top layers come and go, nothing is really being changed by just stripping the layers off earlier than they would usually go naturally

Deeper peels can, in some cases, take up to two weeks to heal. Personally, I can't see how this can be a sensible thing to do to the skin. This is how that whole *Phantom of the Opera* thing started, isn't it? People running around chucking acid on other people's faces?

A too-potent skin peel causes severe blistering, scarring, and a whitening or darkening of the skin. This nasty attack on the skin, this peeling and scraping and scrubbing, is kind of weird and over the top. Naomi Wolf pointed out in *The Beauty Myth* that Clinique says, "Do it as aggressively as possible." But leave some steel wool for the dishes?

Again women are supposed to submit to pain as some kind of duty.

Secret advertising A Melbourne dermatologist explains how this works: "Week after week manufacturers' claims, accompanied by glossy photographs, land on the desks of beauty editors around the world. These heavily biased, subjective blurbs, with the photographs captioned, then appear unedited in the magazines as virtually unpaid advertisements masquerading as independent editorial copy." This is cheap for the magazine and even cheaper for the companies. The only losers are those of us who expect a more critical analysis and those who believe every-thing they read. Now that you know this, you can cast a much more critical eye over the "new products" columns, the beauty stories, the make-overs, and your local newspaper 's ads for beauty salons and weight treatments as well.

APHRODITE, GODDESS of YOU BEAUTY...

KAZ

General fibbing One reason why flashy moisturisers cost 20 times as much as sorbolene cream is not the expensive ingredients but the amount spent in advertising that the company has to make back in sales.

You know the paid, glossy cosmetics advertisements, usually the most expensive full-page, right-hand-side ads in the women's magazines? And the primetime TV ads? Dermatologists are especially concerned that the advertisements suggest that "damage"—from the sun or ageing—can be reversed. This is a lie.

Several U.S. companies have been fined over prattling on fallaciously (that's fibbing) about what their products could do. Effeto Immediato Spa Lift for Face, manufacturer Princess Marcella Borghese claimed, was "formulated with the revolutionary 'Involctin Protein Complex' and the Aqua de Vita 'Living Water' Complex [and] it works to replace skin's natural source of firmness." *Ms.* magazine revealed that the only active ingredient in the $40 bottle was sunscreen.

Legal lies In Australia, essentially, cosmetics ads can get away with lying about what the creams can do, but not about what's *in* the product. In 1990, a spokesperson for the Australian Trade Practices Commission put it this way: "They can say you'll be radiantly lovely and men will goggle at you if you use their products but if they say they contain crushed iguana nostrils they had better contain crushed iguana nostrils."

In America, the Federal Trade Commission can prosecute a company for misleading or deceptive advertising claims. It may investigate outrageous claims such as "slows the aging process," but only on complaint from a consumer, a competitor, or an agency such as the FDA.

Lesley Fair, a senior attorney with the FTC's advertising practices division, said, "Obviously there is some amount of puffery with ads promising 'a more youthful, dewy complexion' or 'more kissable lips' but there are more scientific claims now about protection from photoaging, wrinkle removal and so on. If you say a product

will increase skin moisture by 40 percent you must have independent, verifiable, scientific proof that it really does."

Science fibbing Sometimes it seems you need a degree in scientific language to translate some of these ads. But apparently , this is actually a handicap. "Essentially none of this stuff works," according to a spokesperson for dermatologists. "[Ads are] deliberately written in a pseudo-scientific fashion and the more you know about science the harder it is to make out what they 're saying."

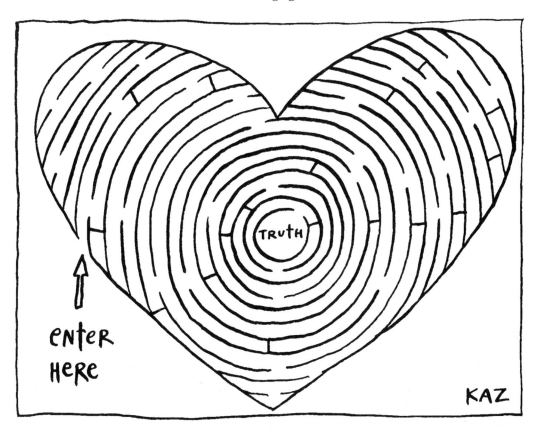

Nivea asks, "Isn't technology beautiful?" and says its double-layer liposomes (fats, remember) deliver "precious moisture." The "Ponds Institute" in TV ads is staffed by languid women in white coats. Clinique is proud of its skin analysis "computer," which is really just a dinky wee plastic thingy with knobs on it. Check one out on a cosmetics counter at a department store near you. They might as well do you a drawing on the back of a paper bag with a stubby old eyebrow pencil.

Elizabeth Arden's "Ceramide Time Complex Capsules... Phenomenon" is pictured like a flying saucer in space, quite near Neptune by the look of things. It is said that this boosts the skin hydration level up to 450 percent after an hour (and wastes a lot of individual plastic in the capsules). That 450 percent, while sounding humungous, would not be visible to the naked eye, so you couldn't tell the difference.

Exolift is actually a piece of sticky tape pressed onto the skin and then removed, carrying dead cells with it (available from "Mediderm"). The International Skin Care Agency claims to be up to their elbows in "phytobiology: the perfect balance of natural aromatic essences, plant extracts and essential oil constituents for - mulated by a French biologist" (thank God he wasn't African or Tasmanian!).

Dior's Svelte is a "new scientific conquest by the Christian Dior laboratories," and is claimed to have "anti-cellulite activity...the silhouette [is] liberated and transformed...a true revolution, proven by tests performed under medical control." Whose control? What tests? Has my silhouette been detained somewhere? Does Amnesty International know about this?

A cosmetics counter saleswoman shows customers a "diagram" of a "plant extract liposome" being swallowed by a skin cell. Dermatologists says this is impossible. Fat molecules and collagen molecules cannot *enter* cells. They're way too big. Try to imagine get - ting your kitchen table down the sink plughole and you'll get the picture.

French fibbing My favourite cosmetics ads are the ones that blather on in French. Even the exported goods from France only for overseas sales have the names in French still on them. In the *Addams Family* television show and movies, when Morticia speaks French her husband, Gomez, swoons with desire and starts kissing her arms. French names in advertising are supposed to have a similar effect on us.

Why say "concentrated gel" when you can say "Gel Concentré Multi-Actif "? Doesn't "Eclat de Jeunesse" sound less unlikely than "burst of youth"? And "Buste Galbe et F ermeté" more sophisticated than "bust shape and firmness"? You can get respect, serenity , balance, and curves in a bottle and it all sounds more plausible in French—*estime, serenissime, harmonie,* and *galbes.* What a load of *merde.*

Environmental hazards At a recent seminar on women's health and the environment in North America, the conference was told that seemingly unrelated problems, from cancer to menstrual disorders, infertility and chronic fatigue syndrome, often resulted from women's unique susceptibility to environmental poisons such as pesticides and lead.

It was reported that the essential female hormone estrogen is vulnerable to such poisoning. Breast cancer has been linked to a higher concentration of DDT pesticides and other organochlorins in the blood. Women in the petroleum and chemical industries have a higher rate of breast cancer.

In the face of a poisoned earth, all the cosmetics companies suggest to tackle the problem is spreading more fat on your face.

Estée Lauder claims that its Advanced Night Repair Protective Recovery Complex will "help prevent environmental damage: ultraviolet rays and free radicals." Free radicals are unstable molecules—feral sciencey things that the skin produces when it is exposed to sunlight or pollution. Free radicals run amok and break down the elasticity of the skin.

Clarins' Power Moisturiser claims "the power of environmental protection. Safeguard skin's beauty from the visible effects of environmental aggression and air pollution." Monteil's Ice Monteil moisturiser "intercepts skin-damaging 'toxic hazards' before ageing effects begin to show." Odélys promises to help with "stress, pollution and the hectic pace of modern living" with plant and marine extracts.

Bioelements has a product called Urban Detox. *Elle* magazine claimed on its behalf that "it protects skin from dangerous environmental hazards while it neutralises the formation of free radicals that lead to premature ageing."

If we continue to give more priority to our skin care than to our planet care, we're going to have a worse environment and worse skin, because it absolutely can't be fixed once it's damaged (that's the skin, not the planet).

The brainy briny "Marine technologies," which usually turns out to mean seaweed or plankton, mud (it's called *fange* in France, chérie), or just plain old seawater are other miracle cosmetic ingredients that pop up now and then. *Diet and Lifestyle* magazine practically wet itself about seawater. "It's naturally alive, containing living organisms, which have a self-purifying and rejuvenating power." Not to mention anchovies, squid, and, in selected world locations, oil spills. All this may make you feel good, but again, there's no evidence of skin penetration benefits.

This didn't stop *Mademoiselle* magazine from prattling, "According to our skin-care forecast, a new wave of seaweed-based products may help fight acne, fend off wrinkles, even block sun damage." The sources for the story included the president and founder of a company selling the first seaweed-based skin-care line, a vice-president of research and development at Estée Lauder, and (ha, now we're getting somewhere!) a vice-president of "creative marketing" for Revlon.

Cleansers Plain, unscented soap and water will do—honest. Cosmetics industry research shows that their fancy claims about special cleansing lotions have been ignored by the 70 per-cent of women who still use soap and water to clean their faces. Accordingly, the companies now flog soaps that make the same claims as the lotions. Or they say you need special moisturising to counter the drying effect of the soap. (Only un-usually dry skins should not be washed with soap.)

Toning Guess what? Toners are completely unnecessary, a con. Many toners contain alcohol and, like aftershaves, they are supposed to constrict the pores after cleansing and before moisturising. "Toning is basically a waste of time and money. The products...basically consist of water , alcohol and glycerine," sums up one dermatologist. The only thing a toner might usefully do is help remove detergents from washing with soap, but a good rinse with water does that too. All a toner will do is make you feel pampered. What toners do very well is look pretty -pretty in their artificial colours of pink and blue, often in sexy, curvaceous designer bottles (a lot more curvaceous than they say we should be).

Exfoliation This means sloughing off dead skin cells, speeding up a natural process. Various scrubs are available. A gentle wash-cloth with soap and water will do a lot of it. Companies will try and sell you volcanic mud, apricot seeds, and everything else short of driveway gravel for the job.

Hypo-allergenic cosmetics This means designed for sensitive skins, so not carrying extra fragrances and colours. Some people confuse it with "hyper -allergenic," thinking it is likely to cause allergic reactions. A hypo-allergenic product doesn't guarantee you will not be allergic to it.

Drugs "Cosmeceuticals" is the clumsy word being suggested to explain the blurred crossover between drugs and cosmetics. Acids fall into this category because they change the structure and/ or function of a part of the body. Cosmetics companies are not registering these as drugs and some say this is because they would then be subject to greater scrutiny and regulation about testing, distribution, and advertising.

Safety labelling The long-term effects of many products are simply unknown but cosmetics now must be labelled under guidelines by the Food and Drug Administration. The label must include a list of all ingredients (but not the quantities), so people can check for anything they're allergic to. Pamphlets must be available at point of sale for items too small for a label, such as lipstick. But according to one pharmacist, "That doesn't help you or me very much because you need a degree in organic chemistry to understand what the compounds are."

On average, a lipstick wearer will swallow 10 pounds of lipstick over 40 years, says the head of toxicology at a Sydney hospital. He worries that of more than 10,000 chemicals used in cosmetics, only about 500 have been tested. " For too long people have assumed that cosmetics are harmless and that they simply sit on the skin. We now know that a lot of people absorb a lot of drugs through their skin."

Urocanic acid in sunscreens was shown to affect the immune system and was linked with cancer in mice during tests at Sydney University, which saw an increase in tumours among rats treated with the acid and exposed to ultraviolet light. There was an Australian recall of the products containing urocanic acid in 1990, including self-tanning products, moisturisers, and makeup from Avon, Clarins, Clinique, Estée Lauder, and Shiseido.

Dermatologists say allergic reactions are rare but consumers need the detailed labelling to protect themselves.

Nature and nurture Some newer companies are producing "natural" cosmetics. These products have feel-good, smell-good components such as essential oils, non-animal soaps, and vegetable and plant extracts. Many also have chemical preservatives. Some herbal products are very expensive for no obvious reason, and some people are allergic to natural substances.

Most of the "natural" products avoid animal extracts, which means (don't read on if you're a queasy type) you miss out on ambergris (from whales) and dried beaver's genitals in perfumes; collagen (animal tissue) and hyaluronic acid (from roosters' combs) in moisturisers; estrogen (from pregnant horse's pee); tallow (animal fat) in soap, lipstick, and shampoos; and spermaceti (more poor whaley bits) in creams and shampoos. Sometimes these will be given alternative scientific names to further disguise their ancestry.

Clarins advertises geranium, ivy, aloe, lavender, mint, and many more yummy-sounding things without saying exactly what they are supposed to do apart from being "natural." The Skin Firming Concentrate has horsetail, horse chestnut, pineapple, and condurango, which I previously had pegged as a Peruvian dissident's club. Egg white and gelatin are also used in many moisturisers because they tighten the skin until they are washed off again.

Did you ever imagine something called hyaluronic acid was from roosters' combs? I guess "New improved dead chicken parts in a can!" doesn't quite have the same allure.

Further information

Your local pharmacist will tell you about cheap moisturizing cream. Be careful when buying books about natural or do-it-yourself beauty products—not all the ingredients are readily available. We don't want you going out on a fruitless search for worzelroot and haunchpoot.

Makeup

Going without vs. getting slathered All the women we have presented to us as role models are wearing makeup—in magazines, in films, on television. A large proportion of the makeup industry is even structured around buying expensive makeup which will not look like makeup—an artifice to cover blemishes and variations, and the perverse "natural"-coloured lipstick.

We are told that without makeup we look tired, washed out, we are not making the effort; we feel, even, that we "haven't got our face on." Women are not supposed to look tired or strung out or sick or in trouble. All things that show up in a face and can be masked by makeup. These real emotions and afflictions must be hidden and unacknowledged. We must pretend. Put on a happy face.

Don't expect magazines to tell you that your face is better off breathing without makeup, or that the no-makeup look is perfectly fine. Their advertisers would have a *fit*. Or possibly kittens.

The makeup sellers and the magazines in their thrall have done very well in turning around the public image of makeup. Before the 1920s, a woman openly wearing makeup was likely to be shunned from "polite" society as a strumpet (what a great word).

When you're just becoming a teenager, the world of *Seventeen* and *Sassy* magazines seems glamorous and mysterious. I learned from them that you couldn't just do nothing to yourself. I learned that there was, in fact, an exhaustive amount of stuff you had to do to be a teenage girl. Boys could just throw on a T-shirt and walk out the door (although I'm sure a lot of them did air-guitar and hair smoothing and checking for whiskers in front of the mirror) but we had work to do and a lot more products to spend money on. We had to transform ourselves into somebody else. We not only had to "make the effort." We had to be seen to make the effort.

Ask anyone who has come out the other side of adolescence if they'd go back and do it again and the only takers would be deeply insane. It's a time of vulnerability, change, groping around for an identity and a sexuality. At a deeply impressionable time, when all you want to do is be over it and be an adult, one of the lessons of how to be an adult that girls learn is to wear makeup. At a time of being at best radiantly crabby, the messages tell us that if we looked better, we'd feel better.

Even a little girl learns by watching the world around her that putting on makeup is what grown-up women do. When she plays dress-up she puts on some lipstick and clomps around in some high-heeled shoes that are too big for her. This is what she first is taught about what it is to be a woman. And she has learned it from observing us.

A fAbuLoUs MaKe-oVeR!

BefoRe   AfTeR

Makeup can be heaps of fun but it's not compulsory.

Essentially confused "What could be worse than finding you've left your makeup bag at home?" asks an Australian *Fashion Quarterly* journalist, who has obviously never been baled up at the mailbox by three rabid Rottweilers and an ex-boyfriend asking for a $1,000 loan.

The article continues, "Suddenly that nondescript but morale-boosting bag of powders and creams seems to hold the key to your true identity. In fact, it's hard to imagine how you will get through the day without it. Every woman totes around a makeup bag of essential items to cover any kind of emergency, from simple re-

After tHAt

I still remember a day a week into my first office job when I came into work without foundation on. My dress was neat and clean, my hair tidy, and I felt presentable in an office. I was told by my boss that I was not to come into the office without make-up on. I remember feeling insulted and that my face without make-up was my personal choice, but of course being young and inexperienced agreed to the request. I don't any more. What made the situation worse as far as I'm concerned is that my boss was a female.

Delys, 24

touch jobs to a complete overhaul after a workout at the gym. For most people, a blusher is essential..."— and on and on it goes.

This is often the problem with beauty editors and writers. Because of the world they live in, they get convinced of a few things. You can't be beautiful without "product" unless you're a supermodel. Your identity is in a bag. An eyebrow brush is essential. Ha. They actually seem unaware that many women never use blusher; that some use it only at night for big events; that some of us carry only a lipstick on a night out and nothing at all during the day. They have bought the hype from the companies that buy advertising to pay their salaries.

Part of the hype suggests that there is no natural beauty without minimalist makeup foundation and translucent powder and "nude" lipstick and tortured eyebrows. The sections called "beauty " are about selling. The word "beauty " has been, um, slightly hijacked. It's all a bit confusing in the magazines, really, when dangerous diet suggestions might be found under "health" and boxing as a good exercise idea under "beauty."

Beauty pages You know the beauty pages in glossy magazines? Where they run photos of new products and a little paragraph on each one? This is not because the beauty editors have been scouring the shops, getting products independently tested, and deciding which ones are the best to recommend. It's because press releases and free samples arrive at the office all day long. And very often, the paragraph about the product is just exactly word for word what the manufacturer says about it in the press release.

There is no questioning of the claims, no matter how confusing. "Guerlain's Protective Base for the Eyelids is like a mini-foundation and powder-in-one for the eye area, allowing makeup to slide on more easily, and fixing it in place." Say what?

Or "These three colours are set to become classics. Sold as singles, they also blend together brilliantly," says a beauty page about pink, brown, and blue eyeshadows. Blend blue and pink for purple and that losing boxer look! Or blend blue and brown for that kind of muddy, erky look!

And the beauty page is often dominated by a misleading photograph of a model from the magazine's files who isn't wear -ing one single scrap of any of the makeup on the page. Or it might be a photograph supplied by the makeup company. Either way it has been professionally lit, photographed, and made-up.

> I didn't know how to talk to males. I would pack on the make-up to try and make an impression makeup for me was also a face to hide behind. I started to make male friends and now talk to most as I would a female friend. And for the record I wear very little make-up now—and my skin is benefiting from the change! It would take me up to one and a half hours to get ready in the morning. It now takes me less than half the time.
>
> Sandy, 19

And now magazines are crediting the *perfume* the model is supposedly wearing. In a photograph. What next? "And Juniper is also wearing a Tampax tampon for heavy-flow days." Anyway, beauty pages are not critical (in the true sense of the word), or analytical, or questioning, or, most often, anything but unpaid ads.

So too are the "make-over" stories: often with similar cheating on what products are actually used and how exclusively. And the "new beauty looks" articles, with pretend history lessons like, "Not since the 1950s has eyeliner been so important," and recommendation of what colours are in fashion. The "after" photographs are usually better lit with the guinea pig smiling.

And guess what? It's not all on the beauty pages either but escaped and running amok through the rest of the magazine. When the atrocious Australian *Hair, Body and Beauty* magazine ran a story called "Beauty Hints for Flirts" it mentioned no fewer than 27 specific products, not to mention suggesting that you practise flirting with your father. (Oh puh-*lease*.)

Candies What is irresistible about the beauty pages is the way they mash up the lipsticks and shake out the coloured powders and scribble with the lipliners and squish the eye paint around. Doesn't it all look scrumptious? I love this part. I think because I just love paints and crayons and gorgeous colours. I'm not sure it would look so attractive if it were not spilled artistically over a glowing light box but all over my bathroom instead. Then it would be an overpriced mess.

But ahhhh, in the magazines! All art-directed and enticing! It's like a whole lot of glorious candies. Good enough to eat but pretty enough just to look at in those pretty jars, or all right, I admit it, smushed all over the light box.

Despite the fact that *Glamour* magazine makeup survey

> Wearing make-up is asking for approval. Wearing make-up is an apology for our actual faces. Wearing make-up makes it seem as if a woman has something to hide. Wearing make-up makes a woman look older than she actually is.
>
> Writer Cynthia Heimel

results of April 1993 showed that women want less packaging in cosmetics (as well as better sales help, more samples, privacy at the counter, sunscreens, and no animal testing), our choices are still influenced by product packaging. Some women put their plain generic cream into designer bottles, sneaky old thangs.

Trends Ignore all trends in makeup. Otherwise you would be a true fashion victim with a pastel look and false eyelashes one minute, the minimalist (strangely expensive) look the next, and then the full-on accident in a blusher factory caricature. You'll be spending $20 on a Chanel Brilliant Soleil Sheer Lipstick. That's $20 for the no-lipstick look! You could get the same effect with Vaseline, one suspects. Or buying waterproof mascara which is rarely anything like waterproof; sometimes it's barely blinkproof. (And beware of mascara without enough preservative in it or old mascara you find under the car seat or in the cutlery drawer. The resultant bacteria can cause permanent eye damage.) Find what you like and experiment without costing yourself a fortune.

The snake pit Rather than rush out and buy all the stuff, take a trip to the nearest mall and try on the testers—being very careful about allergies and transferred germs, of course. This can be fun. But remember the women behind the counter are aliens. They are robots at the front line of the most cutthroat high-markup phenomenal profit business there is.

The cosmetics and perfume

> *Magazine editor at meeting to decide what is going in a women's magazine*: "Right, beauty, and make it quick."
>
> *Beauty editor*: "Clarins, Shiseido, Paloma Picasso, Chanel, makeup, Germolene, lipsticks, powder bases, faces, eyes, lips, nostrils. This is all off the top of my head. Douching with mint is a thought. Ten tips for tropical toenails. I'm thinking natural zing. Moist is my word *de jour*. Skin is in. Lovely wet, moist lips. Wet droplets. Sun, sea, sand, water, waves, beach. I see a photo shoot. I'm looking at two weeks in the Caribbean. And the usual—try and be more beautiful if you want to have more sex."
>
> From *Absolutely Fabulous* by Jennifer Saunders

counters in department stores are known in the trade as the snake pit. These women will lie, insult you gently, undermine your confidence, and put disquieting names to problems you never knew you had because they're not problems. Be careful that instead of letting you play with the paints for fun, they don't turn you into a quivering mass of melting self-esteem, obsessed with pore size (it's genetic and NOTHING sold changes it), eyebrow shape, lipliner, and the like.

Some of those women work on a commission so they get more money for everything they convince you to buy. Others, of course, are darlings and will whisper that you can get a cheaper version at the counter over there which actually works better. Or they will trick you by being nice and saying you have lovely skin you don't need any of these but your eyes might as well be in Poland for all I can see of them, try this divine mascara and let me just cover up your whole face and obliterate your whole identity now hold still or else.

Make a pact with a friend that you will each buy only one thing after testing lots of them and make each other stick to it. Don't forget that you're mostly paying for packaging, which accounts for 60 percent of the price, and the advertising, as well as the salary of this woman standing there trying to look like your skin is the most tragic thing since the invasion of Panama. Or they'll make you "over" and tell you that orange tones are absolutely adorable on you. This is bound to be a filthy lie.

It's always harder for you girls in the country but think of all the money you're saving. And don't forget that while city girls are pay - ing for the expensive big-name brands, your closest pharmacist sells the same stuff, the same shades, only cheaper in different packaging. Avoid those bulk mail orders of lots of cosmetics: why let somebody else choose for you?

Blusher Before Elizabeth Arden Coral Coquette Luxury Cheek Colour and its other modern counterparts, women would pinch their cheeks to bring colour into them. You may be naturally pale, or you may not be getting enough good food for a naturally rosy glow. Most blusher looks fake, unless it's lit and photographed by a professional.

Anyway, the real thing is so awful—I mean blushing. You know, going red and then everyone notices and you can't stop going red, and I'm going red just writing this remembering the other times I've gone red and even my ears went red and the times I've gone red and I haven't even been embarrassed I've been furious or confused or embarrassed for somebody else. Aaaaarrgghhhh! It's feeling, as one friend says, like a caged beet.

And yet here we are buying this product called blusher. It's a hangover from "blushing bride" and other old-fashioned notions of girls kept in the dark about sexual or important matters and "blushing prettily" to show their innocence and girlhood. Bleuuugh.

Eyes Although there is virtually no regulation of the cosmetics industry in the United States, the Food and Drug Administration has warned against the use of eyebrow and eyelash dyes, saying "there is a risk of severe eye injury and even blindness." Even vegetable dyes can cause allergic reactions.

A letter to a problem page I read in a waiting room had a sad letter from a woman who had gone one step further and had her eyebrows tattooed blue-black. One was higher than the other one, and a different shade, giving her a very bizarre permanent expression she couldn't do much about.

Don't buy the mascaras with extra filaments or bits to "extend" or "add to" lashes. You might end up trying to fish them out of your eyes all day. And what exactly is the point of the "no colour" mascara? You might as well just comb your own eyelashes.

Animal testing Companies that claim to have eliminated animal testing themselves can't guarantee that the chemicals they buy have not already been tested on animals.

The phrase "cruelty-free" or "not tested on animals" may mean only that the end product was not tested although each ingredient was.

Some companies use no new ingredients, choosing instead only from a 1978 European Economic Community list of proven safe ingredients. This means these companies cannot advertise amazing new breakthroughs or gobsmackingly sudden age-thwarting inventions. Since 1989, when their safety was established, the Body Shop has used only ingredients that have not been tested on animals.

If you want to be as sure as possible that your cosmetics are made by companies that have genuinely tried to minimise their testing on animals, you can get a list from the Humane Society of the United States, which lists all companies that do no animal testing during the development of or on the finished product. The list also has shampoos and conditioners.

The other way to avoid animal testing is to stick with old favourites from the list and not be lured by the newer products.

Good enough to eat Makeup colours are often named after foods. Forbidden to enjoy eating, women can have guilt-free Raisin (Clinique lip pencil), Rose Chocolat (Lancôme lipstick),

Cherries in the Snow (Revlon lipstick), and a heap of caffeine kickstarters such as Mocha Dream and Cafe Au Lait.

A poll of *Mademoiselle* magazine staff and their favourite cosmetics produced a clear bias in favour of food names. One U.S. company is kicking against the trend with names like "Road-Kill," but it won't catch on. Leatrice Eiseman, of the avoidable-sounding Eiseman Center of Color Information and Training in the U.S. says, "A woman is more likely to buy and stay loyal to a Claret Red for example, than she is to a Number 12."

Lipstick Lipstick is the most common single cosmetic purchase. Most lipsticks are weighted to make it seem as if we're getting more for our money.

Hold just the lid of a lipstick in the palm of your hand and feel how light it is. Now feel the heavier base. The lipstick itself is very light, so you're paying for that extra weighting and packaging. The matte lipsticks have stronger colour. The gloss lipsticks are less drying. There are names like All Day Torrid Perfect Lipstick and New Geranium Luxury Lipstick, Golden Raisin Different Lipstick (pardon?), Café Chic Luxury Lipstick, and even Anger. I am waiting for one called Torrid Crabby Luxurious Raisin Restaurant.

Further information

A full list of preferred products is available from The Humane Society of the United States, 2100 L Street, NW, Washington, D.C. 20037. Include a stamped self-addressed envelope to receive the list. Phone: (202)452-1100. Some of the better-known preferred product makeup brands include Beauty Without Cruelty, Blackmores, Avon, Estée Lauder, Revlon, and the Body Shop. Many other companies are approved for other skin lotions, toothpastes, soaps, cleaning products, sunscreens, pet stuff, and hair products.

Beauty Salons

A little luxury These are little offices we go to when we want to be pampered. They should not be torture chambers and we should not be expected to be transformed by them. For that we need a pumpkin and some mice.

Perfume

Pricey sniffs The first known perfume factory was run by priests in sixteenth-century Italy to help Europeans cover up the fact that personal hygiene had yet to be discovered. Back then, most people never washed themselves. (I'm sorry. These are facts. No wonder they all got the Black Plague. Probably Black Plaque as well.) By 1900, bathing was more common. But more like once a week for the "civilised" world (England, if you don't mind).

Queen Elizabeth I, after all, had announced that she had a bath once a month "whether she needed it or not," and the eleventh Duke of Norfolk only ever had a wash when he got so drunk he passed out, whereupon the poor servants would give him a right going over with a scrubbing brush.

Perfumes in the early part of the twentieth century were considered only for "fast" girls, which is to say girls who like to have a good time. Having a good time and admitting to liking it was considered MOST unladylike. But the first deodorant did not go on sale until the 1920s, so the richer, crabbier women decided that eau de cologne, a watered-down version of perfume which took after its forerunner 4711, which has been around since the 1800s, was acceptable.

Essential oils are now popular, marketed as cruelty-free, without musk (from deer glands), ambergris (bits of endangered whale), or chemicals. Like any other compound, essential oils can cause allergic reactions. They can be used in burners, or on light globes to make a room or house fragrant, rather than a person. Many home-produced body lotions and bubble baths sold in boutiques and at markets are now being made with essential oils and marketed as natural or aromatherapy products.

Aromatherapy is based on the principle that certain scents will induce or encourage different feelings or emotional states: in which case, as I once overheard in a health-food shop, "They should aerial-spray the whole country with lavender so everybody can calm down."

Perfumes can often cause an allergic reaction, particularly if worn in the sun, as this can cause chemicals to react differently with the skin. This is more common with citrus-based scents than others.

Perfume extract is usually 20 to 25 percent perfume essence in 90 to 95 proof alcohol. Eau de toilette is 5 to 8 percent essence diluted in 80 to 90 proof alcohol. The perfume may cost ten times as much but be only three times more concentrated. But you may use more eau de toilette to get the smell level up.

Have you ever been stuck in an elevator or on a bus with somebody who uses too much perfume or aftershave? It's because they become immune to the strong smell, incorporating it into their senses without smelling it themselves. So they build up to putting more and more perfume on every day until the rest of us fall to the floor pleading for mercy, or at least some *air*.

A perfume's price takes into account the cost of ingredients, research and development, exclusivity, design, packaging, advertising, distribution, designer name, and what people will be prepared to pay. (Snobbery is the original aromatherapy.) Advertising campaigns now run into the millions for a single perfume.

Even perfumes that are not heavily advertised or that don't need a launch can chew through the bucks. According to one documentary, a $48 bottle of Chanel No. 5 perfume (which was the same cost per ounce as gold at the time) is worth about $2.25 in ingredients. The rest is money added by administration costs, packaging, advertising, and profit.

Stinko bizarro Perfume must be one of the hardest things to sell. I already like it, but which to buy? All I want is a perfume that smells exactly like a fresh, trembling tuberose but what I get is pictures of Elizabeth Taylor looking as if she's totally lost her marbles, 11-year-old girls poncing around in evening gowns with velvet trains, women (who look as if they're struggling with an eating disorder as well as a dirty great bit of kelp) writhing at the water's edge, a young woman with feathers coming out of her butt wearing a leg leash, a man lurking around with a bunch of peonies, pictures of one naked person giving another one a firefighter's lift, very many pictures of women looking wistfully air-headed surrounded by baskets of floristry, and a whole lot of absolute crap written to describe a scent.

Magazines now carry perfume samples, and American magazines carry up to three separate perfume samples as part of the full-page advertising. (In America you don't need to buy perfume. You just slink up to a newsstand and rub yourself against page 57 of something.)

Perfume is a mega-million-dollar business. Here in the United States they're squabbling over sales worth $2.9 billion. So the companies spend up on their launches of new scents. The perfume companies have monstrously lavish cocktail parties, dinners and parties with fireworks and caviar and obsequious waiters and lots of alcohol and free samples. They invite their closest personal friends: the Press.

After all, advertisers are flogging a wee bit of luxury for the people who can't afford to get invited to the perfume launch parties with caviar and fireworks and *marvellous* old Oscar de la Thingie flown out from (gasp, swoon, stagger) Paris! A bit of romance and glamour in a beautiful bottle. And some of the bottles are very beautiful, delicate, mysterious, gloriously chunky, designed by surreal artists and marketing geniuses. Others push the point, with fake jewels and golden metal butterflies.

We're buying Diamonds and Rubies from Elizabeth Taylor, and Trésor (Treasure) and Tweed, Lace, White Satin, and White Linen that we can't afford to buy or wear because we live in the real world where white linen is impractical. We're buying the sexy, the forbidden, the racy, Volupté, Poison, Tabu, Joy, and Opium (which was banned in Queensland, Australia, for two years). We want to be Knowing, Clandestine, Spellbound, Unforgettable, Beautiful, a Diva, a Paradox; to have Worth, Youth Dew, Mystery, and Panache. We want to associate with a lifestyle: be Miss Dior, be in Paris, or more specifically one of its neighbourhoods, Rive Gauche, or smell of its old money, called Chanel Number 5. We want it for Eternity, Forever. Or at least until 4711.

There are no perfumes called Pre-Menstrual Bitchface or Sheer Poverty.

Hair

It's compulsory Hair: we're covered in it. Although some of it is more luxurious, some is short and curly, and some grows all the time and has to be cut to maintain its length. Other bits don't grow long, which is very handy under the circumstances. I don't fancy an armpit ponytail myself.

Everyone has hair on the

> My major problem would be hair: I have more hair on my arms than my boyfriend. I wax my upper lip and in between my eyebrows and have since I was 13. My current boyfriend made remarks all the time until I broke down and explained that you just don't say those kinds of things to a girl. There are some clothes I will not wear, like bikinis, because I have a little snail trail and a lower hairy back.
>
> Lena, 19

legs, arms, face, and pubic area. In fact, everyone has hair all over
the body. Some have more or darker hair which is more noticeable
on paler skins. We all get hairier as we get older. If your hair feels
dead, it's because it is: all the stuff above the skin surface, anyway.
That's why you can't repair split ends by doing anything except
cutting them off. Eating a balanced diet with protein will make the
hair a healthier corpse. Hair is made from keratin, which is a form
of protein. You can damage your hair with sun, bleach, heat treatments and blow-drying, perms, and chemical dyes. Crash diets and
stress can cause temporary hair loss until you correct the problem.
(Hair loss usually starts two to three months after your nutrition
level drops.)

Hormonal changes at puberty and at menopause can make the
hair oilier. Women on the pill or who are pregnant report that
some perms simply won't take on their hair. Pregnant women have
really shiny hair. And when you go grey is haireditary.

Magazines regularly run stories about "new hair products," some claiming "technological breakthroughs" in shampoo, conditioner, colour, or removal. The last thing they want you to do is leave it alone and stop spending money on your furry bits. And remember, the more you do to your hair, the more you risk damaging it through hea t, chemicals, and harassment.

Getting it off An article in Cosmopolitan warbles on that "re-veal-it-all summer styles call for superbly smooth skin... Summer means lazy days at the beach and as most swimsuits are highcut and revealing, it's time to face that perennial hot weather problem: the abominable bikini line." Or else it's time to face the fact that manufacturers are not producing enough swimsuits with low-cut legs that women want to wear .

Anyway, do you think this article on hair removal has anything to do with the fact that the next page is an ad for Johnson's baby oil and it says "A Johnson and Johnson/*Cosmopolitan* promotion"? And then there's a page called "A *Cosmopolitan* Andrea Promotion" and it's for "Natural Wax Hair Remover." What about the " *Dolly/Waxeeze* Promotion*,*" in which what is basically an ad for hair -removal products is presented like a typical *Dolly* story with the magazine's layout and design style and a file photograph of a model with shorn legs? Let's get this straight. *Dolly* magazine, like all the others, is unlikely to run a whole page of stuff on hair removal unless somebody is directly or indirectly paying for it.

I had my legs waxed for the first time as research for this book. Here are the results: it hurt like hell, my legs felt bald, startled, and affronted, it cost about $20 and would "have" to be done again in a few weeks (oh no, it wouldn't), *plus* it made my legs *itch* like crazy for several weeks afterwards.

Every "expert" and doctor will tell you that hair does not grow back thicker and darker after it has been shaved, waxed, or plucked but women say differently. Many people who fall into shaving away and rigorously plucking out most of their eyebrows, including models, have found that their eyebrows never grow back, or never the same way.

Eyebrows are essential to the look of the face, which is

why drawn-on false ones and plucked-practically -to-oblivion ones look so strange. They change the whole shape of the face and can give you a permanently quizzical, puzzled, and witless expression. If you are determined to change your eyebrows, please don't shave them, not even once just a little bit. Plucking underneath is much less stressful than on the top of the brow. Whether you wax or pluck, it is going to hurt.

There are many ways women remove natural hair. There is shaving, which doesn't last long; waxing, which hurts; depilatory creams (virulent chemicals that dissolve the hair: spooky); electrolysis (in which a needle is poked into each hair follicle at the root of the hair and electrocutes the hair, which falls out and mostly does not grow back), which can leave permanent scarring if not done correctly and can also hurt and is meant to be permanent but sometimes has to be repeated several times on the same follicle; and plucking, which also hurts.

Drugs to make you less hairy can have truly horrifying side effects and, in fact, are very, very rarely needed. Unless you have a history of abnormal menstruation or other symptoms of a hormonal disorder, the amount of hair you have is probably just your natural amount and nothing to do with a medical problem.

Whatever the fashion among your friends, hair removal is not compulsory.

P.S.: Try not to laugh if the person waxing your legs describes herself as an aesthetician.

Further help

If you're worried about a serious condition such as hair loss or major scalp flaking, the American Academy of Dermatology will put you in touch with a trained specialist. It would be safer not to trust a serious problem to a corner hairdresser. The Academy is at 930 North Meacham Road (or P.O. Box 4014), Schaumburg, IL 60168-4014. Phone: (708)330-0230.

When there's a society for the prevention of bossy hairdressers, I will let you know.

chapter six

You are not your buttocks

Self-image and self-esteem

Love the one you're with For a long time women's self-esteem has been tied to their feelings about physical appearance. Women are told not only that "you are what you eat" but that "you are what you look like."

With so much criticism, it can be hard to "love the one you're with."

Health workers have observed that eating behaviour and body image are closely connected. "For women, this connection is deeply related to their self-esteem, as it seems they have always been valued as objects of beauty and desirability...however, this is somewhat different from men who obtain their self-esteem via achievements, power status and control," according to one manual for health workers who are setting up body-image groups.

The manual says what is needed is social change, and "educating women to explore their own body shape and what's comfortable and healthy for them, and alerting them to the social and economic forces so that they too can challenge them...it is about challenging women to value and see themselves as a whole person, and celebrate their body as both decorative and functional."

The Body Image and Eating Behaviour Project, led by community nurse Penelope Goward and run by the Victorian Health Promotion Foundation's Eating Behaviour Unit, identifies that a woman feeling unhappy or worthless will not express herself that way, but instead say, "I'm fat" or "I'm ugly." This grossly distorted view has become "normal" behaviour in

> I have panic attacks about being fat. When I look in the mirror I see a thin/skinny person, but as soon as I walk away I imagine myself as fat. I know what I'm doing, and I chastise myself for being ridiculous, but the paranoia is overwhelming.
>
> Graffiti in Queensland University law faculty women's toilets

women. Instead of decoding the feeling "I am fat" to find that we are feeling unloved, dull, or depressed, many of us just relate it to our body size or shape.

A university study found that in 35 surveyed couples, the women chose significantly thinner photographs to indicate what they thought their partners wanted than those their partners actually chose. A Flinders University study in Adelaide of 92 adults, 78 teenagers, and 71 children showed that women and teenage girls—not men and teenage boys—believed they were larger than they needed to be to appear attractive.

Disturbingly, both the boys and girls aged nine and ten rated their figures as larger than ideal. The researchers concluded that "one can only speculate that the imagery surrounding fatness and slimness as demonstrated on television and through other media is very influential in determining children's beliefs."

Cleo magazine's dieting survey showed that 73 percent of participants envied somebody else's body every day, and that every day more than half of the women felt depressed about their weight. Seventeen percent avoided mirrors altogether. Others saw a distortion in the mirror.

Recent surveys in the United States found that 47 percent of normal-weight women want to be thinner.

Pressure to have bad body image Where do we start?

The censored image of women in TV and film shows only the thin; magazines suggest that body "flaws" should be disguised, dieted against, or exercised away.

Women in lingerie ads are nearly one-quarter thinner than average women, and much taller as well. Even if these models were of average height they could put on 18 to 20 more pounds without causing any health problems. But they are touted as having "the perfect body."

The definition of "the perfect body"—indeed, the idea that there might be only one—has been announced by media commentators who have no right to do so. There is more than one definition of a "good body" or a "fabulous body." A "perfect body" is a myth.

Body hatred is fashionable. Young girls watch adult women, and they know that one of the ways to be a big girl, a grown-up, is that we have to grab hold of a part of ourselves with disgust and say, "Look at this, I'm too fat." Everyone else says, "No you're not, I am. Look at this! Feel this!" grasping bits of themselves. Part of being a woman is projected as specific self-loathing in the face of evidence to the con-

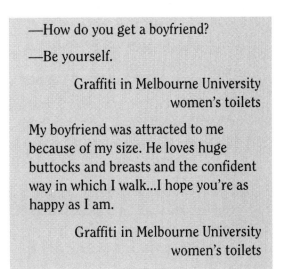

—How do you get a boyfriend?

—Be yourself.

Graffiti in Melbourne University women's toilets

My boyfriend was attracted to me because of my size. He loves huge buttocks and breasts and the confident way in which I walk...I hope you're as happy as I am.

Graffiti in Melbourne University women's toilets

trary. Anybody observing can see that the flesh being grabbed is not too fat. And still the self-definition insists: the distortion is lore, and law.

At only 93 pounds, 1960s model icon Twiggy said she "hated what I looked like...I ate like a horse and just burned off everything. Like most skinny people, I desperately wanted to put on weight."

Being thin Thin women are not immune from body hatred and bad self-image and self-esteem. Thin girls are taunted about being bony and skinny and not having prominent breasts. Nasty comments are made questioning their femininity, their warmth as human beings, and whether they have an eating disorder. There are rude, envious comments: "You're such a bitch, you're so thin." One thin woman, writing of her experience in a newspaper, said, "There are many garments the thin female shouldn't wear. Like clothes that expose just about any part of the body...not a pretty sight. Would the old chook who is exposing her horrible scrawny knees on the cocktail party circuit please take note?...When you lose weight the first thing to go are the bosoms, of course...women tend to be flat-chested if their other vital statistics are pared down. Sexy isn't exactly the word for a Skinny Minnie at the beach or in her lingerie." But thin woman are just as sexy as bigger ones, and no less womanly for having smaller curves.

> I spend a lot of time writing letters to readers, particularly the younger ones, repeating the phrase, "If you are within the healthy weight range for your height and are fit, healthy and active, you have every right to be proud of your body." I don't know how many take it to heart though. It's one of those things that's very easy to accept intellectually, but so hard to truly believe...I also find myself writing to people [to tell them] they must put out of their heads the idea that by losing the weight they will automatically look like a fashion model. No amount of dieting is going to make a wide-hipped woman of 4'11" decrease the size of her pelvis and grow 12 inches [in height]. It seems to me that... most of us think if we can get this right, every other aspect of our lives will automatically be perfect.
>
> Diane Parks, Australian editor, *Slimming* magazine

٭♡٭

Just like everybody else In adolescence, the changes in our body are the first real major changes since we started walking and talking. Our families talk about the changes, and maybe they tease us. Kids at school notice development or no development.

We want to shrink into the crowd, be like everybody else, too obsessed and freaked out to notice that everybody else is freaked out and different too. Even those who are teasing us. We read magazines to find out how to be "normal," how to look like everybody else. This is exactly the way to become a dull or scared person: perhaps more likely to be picked on.

꒷♡꒷

Self-esteem and puberty According to a study conducted by the Australian Institute of Sport, which mimics international findings, the self-confidence levels of boy and girl athletes at about ages 13 and 14 are pretty much identical, and after that they drop off, but the female level drops off quicker and to a greater extent than the male level. The study adds, "For both sexes it seems to bottom out or reach its lowest levels at around 19, 20, 21 years of age and then it bounces back out again, but interestingly the males actually end up higher than when they started, and the female athletes never reach the same level [as at 13 and 14] again."

This research suggests that even the female "winners" in our society—the study was of 1,798 athletes over six years to 1989, who were physically fit and still winning—will reach a peak of self-esteem before puberty and never again reach that level as young people or adults.

> Throughout my early teens I did not like myself and thought I was chubby. I look back at photos of myself and see that I was actually quite slim: and in fact slimmer than some of the girls I envied.
>
> Carol, 19

Similar results were found by a 1991 study of 200 ninth-grade students in Sydney called "Adolescents' Problems and Their Relationship to Self-Esteem." Girls' self-esteem declined dramatically at puberty: girls were more concerned about societal and personal relations, courtship, sex, marriage, and physical development. Boys were more concerned about finance, education, and career issues.

The authors of the study said some things became clear

from asking young people what they think: "While the media promotes an image of the physical, personal and interpersonal attributes that girls should attain, it virtually ignores those areas for boys, who are encouraged to become educated, combative and aggressive for personal and economic survival."

Not even my academic achievements can drag me up out of the dumps when I am confronted with...The Mirror! I am confronted almost every day in the mirror at ballet class where the leotards and tights tell everyone about the chocolate I ate at lunch.

Diana, 20

Government education policies acknowledge that girls are inclined to explain their successes by external factors, such as help from parents and teachers and luck, but blame themselves for failures. Boys usually blame failure on bad luck or unfair tests. It seems we could learn something from the boys.

Deborah Saltman, an associate professor of social and preventive medicine at Queensland University, says girls have a lot of trouble with their changing bodies, and can feel "freakish." They also have to come to terms with double standards about their sexuality— they should be sexy-looking, but also be "good girls" without a bad reputation. Dr. Saltman says girls need to know that adolescence is a time of big changes, where you can experiment, make mistakes, and feel whatever it is you're feeling—angry, sad, not like talking, whatever. (Of course, your family will probably think you are a drug addict.)

One of the things I have that slightly cheers me up is a picture of Marilyn Monroe. She's trying on a black bikini and my God, she's absolutely fat and she looks wonderful.

Kim, 23

How to like yourself Psychologist Thomas Cash and graduate student John Buttershave created a body-image therapy which combines body education, relaxation techniques, and guided imagery to change ingrained body-image distortions. Patients are taught to move from "I'm so ugly. Everyone looks better than me" to "I like the way I look. I don't mind people looking at me." Sometimes this takes months. One woman who did the course says she still thinks her thighs and hips are too big, but she doesn't dwell on it and is able to go to beach parties.

Many women's health centres, state health departments, hospitals, and community centres run body-image courses. Body-image groups are usually small—six to eight people—and women only. One women's health centre encourages participants to stop thinking about the body as parts of a machine that need to be controlled, and to think of the whole body. Participants keep a journal and study their inner voices to hear if that's them talking, or society, or somebody else. Attitude to food is also explored, including other experiences that can make you feel rewarded, and nutrition information. Participants learn that their body knows what shape and size it needs to be. You have to listen to what your body really needs: a decent feed and the odd bit of exercise.

Body-image boosters
Come back and read this section any time you feel bad about yourself. Some of the following ideas may be incorporated into a body-image group you decide to attend.

Examine yourself Stand in front of a mirror with no clothes on (lock the door!). You can start with your clothes on the first time if you can't look at your nakedness. Describe yourself out loud or write it down neutrally, as if you were describing a statue or painting. You can do this as you are rubbing in a moisturising cream, perhaps with an aromatherapy fragrance.

Analyse yourself If you think a part of yourself is unacceptable, you must say why. Not "Because it doesn't look good"—why doesn't it? Who said that? Who told you? Why did they say that? Who agrees with them? How do you know? Okay, now you have finished with that. Finished. Get dressed and go away from the mirror. Next time, get undressed, lock the door. Look at yourself. List all the positive things about your shape.

Live happily in your body Some ways of feeling that your whole body is you, and not just a whole lot of bits latched onto you like carpet fluff, include doing regular exercise such as swimming, walking, or yoga. I know I always feel better about my body, lighter and more together, after I do yoga. Yep, those three mornings a year I remember to do my yoga are always truly great. Other postural and movement disciplines, including the Alexander technique and dancing (not ballet or gym or anywhere else where they panic about their weight), can be useful. A young woman who took belly-dancing lessons said, "Through the dance, my body expresses itself in ways I haven't heard before, the lumps and bumps get a chance to speak. It's like a body language. My legs are heavy for my size but in dance they are supportive." The other girls and women from the class said dancing together had given them a more realistic image of women's bodies.

Exercise In general, fit and healthy people feel better about themselves. People who take care of themselves (thanks, but no more unprocessed whale lard for me and I don't think I will have that fourteenth tequila slammer) can find they have a corresponding realisation that they are worth caring about. This is not the false "caring about yourself" that involves things like depriving yourself of food and overexercising, or wearing makeup but not having that changing mole checked, or ironing your clothes but having sex without a condom.

Analyse messages Every time you see a magazine article telling you to be thinner, exercise more, or wear more flattering clothes, don't let it hang like a personal accusation. Ask first: Why is the magazine running this story? To sell clothes, to sell cosmetics? Because they believe it? Because they're too scared to stop? Because they know we're all interested in body image and they know their story on it, positive or negative, will boost sales? Why should I listen to this? What will happen if I reject this idea? What will happen if I recycle this magazine and go and have a Twinkie?

Reward yourself Choose a variety of treats, not just food—bubble baths, girls' nights out, holidays, congratulations, a new book, red shoes, flowers, art, whatever takes your fancy.

Be realistic As Robin Morgan, editor of *Ms.* magazine, says about feminism, "Change doesn't come from the top." Don't expect the magazines to change; they will not, unless we force them. And even then, the advertiser's dollar will be stronger than ours. *Ms.* magazine has no ads for this very reason—so its editorial content will not be influenced by advertising. It has no articles on hair, no weight-loss diets, no cosmetics, no fashion. That's why it costs $5.95.

Describe yourself Body-image experts say it is important for girls to stop seeing their physical selves as "the most important aspect of their whole being." So here's another exercise (and you don't have to do anything like a leg lift). Sit down somewhere quiet and make

real *gorgeous*

a list of all your attributes. Pretend you are describing yourself in minute detail to somebody from another planet you have never met, who will have to guess who you are. You are not allowed to refer to anything physical whatsoever. Make a list of all your positive characteristics and knowledge. Make a list of what your friends like about you. Try describing your friends without making reference to their appearance.

Be a whole person Achieve in other areas, gain control of other areas, so you don't get obsessed with the outside of yourself. This may mean joining a team sport, exploring an artistic pastime, developing an interest in film, photography, nature studies, politics, engineering. Join a rock band, write songs, draw cartoons, act, run, sew, cook, embrace experiences and chances, make jokes. Hang out with people who accept you and like to do things, who don't just sit around talking about bodies, diets, tanning, and obsessing about food. That's boring and passive.

Get to know your body Learn anatomy, have massages, acupressure, foot reflexology. Feel yourself breathing, exercising, relaxing.

Fight the body police Prepare ways to respond to people who feel they can comment on and judge your appearance, even those who think they are being "helpful." (You will find some hints in the body police section at the end of this chapter.)

Clean house Throw away pictures of models you might have cut out or kept in your head that you have aspired to look like. Understand that they are *them* and you are *you*.

Accept your genes Look at different members of your family and family photographs as far back as you can go. Recognise family traits, without judging them as good or bad.

Be a pal When possible, support other women and girls in their body image. I can still remember my aunt saying to me as a teenager, "You have beautiful, strong legs. They're wonderful." I was sceptical but she was obviously sincere, so I was forced to consider what she said. I can also remember a great-aunt saying rudely and dismissively in front of me, about me, but not to me, "She's very *solid* isn't she?" I still love the first aunt, and I wouldn't give you 20 cents for the other one, who was a lot more solid than I was and probably felt better by insulting me. Maybe she didn't think at all, maybe she was just brainwashed.

Analyse your feelings Change the way you talk about yourself from negative to neutral or optimistic phrases. Write down the things you know you have said about yourself and look at other ways of expressing them. For example, "My skin looks disgusting" could become "I am freaked out about my skin." "I look worse than ever" may become "I usually look better than I do now." "I hate my fat hips" translates to "My hips are the widest part of me."

Stand up for your rights Defend the gains women have made in being taken as individuals and recognised for their talents and contributions, not just for what they look like. Support equal opportunity at home and at work and preserve and celebrate the institutions, laws, and people who are still fighting for that equality.

Be a really whole person See your body as your home, the kind thing you live with, in, and as. Not as something separate from you.

Express yourself Put on a tape or the radio and sing. Loud. Really loud. Belt it out. When the neighbours come to complain, explain it's for your self-esteem. See if you can get them to dance. Singing is expressing yourself, an emotional release. Joining a drama group will also help boost self-esteem. If you feel overwhelmed by the awful inner voice telling you that you are too fat, get it out, in poems, drawings, songs, a diary, or a journal. Exercise it and may it be exorcised.

Get smart Psychiatrist James Masterton says there are some keys to improving your self-esteem. Staying flexible about creative solutions to old problems; understanding the difference between who you are and what other people think of you, which "enables you to do what feels right for you, even when others disagree"; and having intimacy with yourself and with others as your real self, without pretence. Recognition of the things you are good at should always accompany your feeling that something did not work, or is not the way you would like it to be. "Accentuate the positive" as the awful song goes.

Be a nature lover Change thinking about the body as something that can be sanitised and tidied: words like *slim* and *trim*, *nip* and *tuck* suggest neatness. Human bodies are not neat. We are the rounded, hairy things.

Choose your media If magazines are bothering you, give them a rest or train yourself to read them more critically. Recognise that one image of woman is regularly praised by magazines, TV, and movies: the woman who tries to please men. The idea that we must please men by our appearance, and that we can be judged by our appearance alone, can be challenged.

Take a compliment Listen to your friends, families, and lovers when they say they love you the way you are. Question the motives of those who don't and plot ways of getting away from their undermining.

Give compliments But ask yourself what kind of compliment you are giving. Are you telling somebody by your actions or conversation that you think they are interesting, worthy, healthy-looking, happier? Or are you saying "You look good because you look thinner": a much more boring and ultimately destructive compliment that says more about your own problems with shapes and sizes than what you think of the other person.

How to find a body-image group

Ask at your local community or women's health centre, the regional or state health department, local hospital, or eating disorders support group for one to join, or start one with their help.

Further reading

Marcia Hutchinson, *Transforming Body Image* (New York: Crossing Press, 1985). Recommended for use with a health professional.

Marion Crook, *The Body Image Trap* (Canada: Self Counsel Press, 1991). Historical and psychosocial look at overeating and body image.

Dr. Judith Rodin, *Body Traps* (New York: Morrow, 1992).

Barry Glassner, *Bodies* (Los Angeles, Lowell House, 1992).

Hara Estroff Morano, *Style Is Not a Size: Looking and Feeling Great in the Body You Have* (New York: Bantam Books, 1991).

Starhawk, *Truth or Dare Encounters with Power, Authority and Mystery* (San Francisco: Harper & Row, 1987). Discusses issues of power and body image.

The body police

Hassled by the body police Families, relatives, and friends feel they have a right to comment on a girl's body when it begins to change at puberty. Girls are taught to expect exposure and commentary and judgement from others, often based on unrealistic ideals. The girls are shamed and turn to dieting and exercise. Body -image expert Penelope Goward also notes this. "If

I loathed mirrors and shopping for clothes. When I was 16 something changed. I discovered the world of performing arts...I left my school to go to a performing arts course in 12th grade. My folks were horrified. They said I could not succeed because I was "fat." I wasn't doing it as a career move, I was doing it to gain confidence in myself. And I did gain confidence, slowly. According to conventional tables I am 88 pounds overweight. I've always had plenty of boyfriends and offers for as long as I have felt confident about myself. I have recently started working as a photographic model and a life-drawing model: confident women of my shape and size are in short supply so I'm getting plenty of work. I still have my "fat days," my "ugly days," and my "bad hair days" but I am generally satisfied with the way I look.

Willa, 24

I hate being skinny. When I get sick I have no reserves and feel so weak and skinny: it's a really scary feeling. I believe there is too much pressure on females to look great. What is inside is much more important. I am finally learning this. Someone who is only average-looking can appear so beautiful—if they are happy and kind on the inside it will make them glow with beauty on the outside.

Mandy, 21

I hate my face because it's too fat. I would much rather be anorexic than obese or overweight. When I look in magazines I think how I'd love to be skinny. Everywhere I look there are skinny people, which makes me hate myself even more. I have tried to commit suicide about four times. I wish magazines would stop portraying "fat" as being bad.

Amy, 16

you have received negative feedback about your body as a child and adolescent, you will have low self-esteem about your body when you grow up."

∴♡∴

How to deal with the body police So many of the girls and women who wrote to me about this book could remember the comment that first started them dieting, and often spurred them on to an eating disorder, especially bulimia.

Perhaps if you show this book to members of your family they will realise the damage their "joking" or judgement may have.

Explain to them they might have forgotten that the natural changes at puberty don't match the pictures of girls and women seen in magazines and on TV. Let them know that their comments—about something you cannot and should not try to control—are training you for food obsessions, eating disorders, and a lifetime of self-loathing. Ask them to accept you the way you are.

At 5'7" tall, weighing around 120 pounds, it hasn't been any easier for me to get dates or a boyfriend, wear clothes that I'd like to, meet more people, wear a bikini with confidence or anything else that "fat" people think we do with ease. What it takes is confidence— confidence to love your body and love who you are.

Amanda, 17

I walked along the beach in the moonlight, looking down at my strong, rounded white legs. I suddenly thought, "I like those legs. They're a bit strangely shaped and wobbly up the top, and they've got me around for 30 years, and dammit, I like them."

Lucy

My boyfriend is only 20 to 30 pounds heavier than myself, but I feel larger than he is. He is also taller. My clothes can be literally falling off me (I am a size 8) and I still feel big and fat.

Annette, 25

Three years ago I put on a little bit of weight and went up to 145 pounds, which is okay. I was informed by my grandparents, sister, and parents that I was "getting fat." I then changed to a gluten- and dairy-product-free diet and exercised like mad. I lost 26 pounds. I was then told I'd lost too much weight. I've been called ugly, beautiful, and pretty, hassled due to my big breasts and hips, called fat, skinny, a rake. What am I supposed to think? The main influence on me in these areas is my family. I am doing nursing and we are educated about positive self-esteem, eating disorders, weight ranges. But somehow, I don't know why, the experts and print media, although (probably) they give more truthful information, do not have the same amount of influence as those we know and the visual media.

Kathleen

One of the marching girls' chaperones exclaimed, "My God you're never going to fit into your uniform, I've never seen anyone grow outward so fast that much." All the girls started calling me "Big Mumma." The tears came to swell in my eyes. Then I decided to only have dinner and starve myself all day and this went on for about a month. I became very moody, pale, and very, very thin. The coach told my mum, she was very concerned but didn't do much about it. One morning I had an aching back. I had a look at it in the mirror and there were bruises all up my spine. I told my coach about it and she said it was the first sign of anorexia. I am now back on my feet and am 5'5" tall and 117 pounds and slowly recovering.

Tanya, 16

If they don't, try to remember that so many parents, especially mothers, have been subjected to the same nasty pressure about bodies and the fear of fat. They can project their fears on to you through comments such as "You're getting fat," even when you are the perfect shape and size for yourself. (Remember that you may have different genes than your mother or sisters.)

You can use this book to show your family that dieting does not work, and that if you eat healthy foods and exercise three times a week for more than half an hour, you are the right size and shape for you. Many people will be surprised at this information because of the diets and propaganda they see on television and in magazines and their own history of struggle with body image. They may not believe you because it is too confronting for them.

As for guys, the young ones who try to torture you with insults and comments are just absolute dickbrains. They are just trying to make themselves feel tougher. How many of them say these things when they are on their own? They don't have the guts or the reason: they have only been trying to impress their mates.

Girls and women who make cruel or thoughtless comments have the same motivation. If they can impress their standards on you, they can feel better about the dieting crap they put themselves through. If they see you are happy with what you are, they feel threatened because they are still trapped by the lies they have been told. They make themselves feel prettier and better by knocking you.

Sure it's fine to please friends and family, but remember you only have one life and you should give yours a little bit more attention... If people do not like what you do or the way you look, it would be the person's problem, not yours. We have to start to realise that there is nothing wrong with ourselves individually and that only people who want to see faults and pick them out are the ones with the abnormality in society. Trying to be accepted by them...robs us of the opportunity of being unique and different to one another. It stops us from who we really want to be and feel comfortable being.

Penny, 17

—I'm skinny. Are you jealous?

—Not at all. I am cuddly and soft. Are you jealous?

—I'm fat and I have a great sex life.

Graffiti in Melbourne University women's toilets

Throughout elementary school and junior high I was the butt of some of the kids' jokes. I had and still have the "big nose syndrome." I would get the teasing, the name calling. It was terribly, terribly hard to ignore. When I got to senior high it ceased, almost. Still there are the totally obnoxious people at parties, that 90 percent of the other people would love to impale on a sharp stick and set fire to. Although I am still very conscious of the bit of me that's unfairly dominant, I have a groovy time.

Irina, 18

"From now on you will not be having cakes or dessert," announced my megalomaniac mother in front of the whole family. I was seven years old, for crying out loud. So I was put on the right track for a lifetime of eating disorders and self-image distortions. By the age of 11 I had reached my adult height. "You could be so good-looking if you weren't so fat. Fat people are ugly. Fat people are psychologically disturbed. Fat people don't get jobs because normal people don't trust them because they think they are greedy. I'm only telling you this because I care about you and I want to protect you from how other people will react. Don't look at cookbooks it will give you bad ideas." I can't believe all of the abuse my parents put me through has had such a lasting effect.

Anonymous, 24

My friend says, "My mum's never happy with me and tells me I need to go on a diet, but it's easy this way [bulimia]." I had just bought a new outfit. All my friends commented on how great...it looked on me and I thought so, too. I couldn't wait to get home and show Mum. To my disappointment this is what my mother said, "Oh it looks great...although you just have to lose weight in your legs first, hey?" Most of my friends just want to please mum and get her approval.

Daisy, 17

I grew up in dancing classes from the age of three and have seen candid close-ups of the pain that girls and women experience when subjected to constant scrutiny about their bodies.

Julie, 20

Older guys who still put pressure on women about their figures are ignorant. If you are with a man who puts you down for who or what you are, you are with the wrong man. If you continue to allow him to dictate your self-esteem, you will spiral down. You may end up being an emotionally or physically abused person, too cowed to know how to get away and find people who will appreciate you for yourself, and men who will think you're gorgeous because they like you. They *are* out there but you won't find them if you stay in situations that reinforce bad feelings about yourself. If he doesn't shape up, ship out. He has the problem, not you.

When you cannot make your family understand, and when the comments come from people at school, at parties, or in the workplace, you may need some help in dealing with the

My best friend started seeing a man who told me on a number of occasions I was overweight and should lose it. I became very self-conscious and went to see a dietitian. By eating sensibly and exercising three times a week I lost around 20 pounds and others said I looked really good. Soon I was eating less and exercising six times a week. I was underweight but could not stop. I weighed myself every morning and thought about being fat at least every five minutes...I was admitted to an eating disorders unit. I was happier fat, but I just can't let go of wanting to be thin and accepted.

Cheryl, 23

If I ever went to my friend Karen's house she and her mother were trying to convince me to do the same as Karen and go on a diet.

Danni, 17

My brother is 15 years old and constantly makes remarks about my figure. If we are having a fight he calls me "thunderthighs" or tells me to lose weight. I play volleyball, touch football, and walk absolutely everywhere I can. At one stage 18 months ago I became very self-conscious about my body and began to vomit up my food. One day I was walking to the train station when a group of about six guys walked past me. One said, "Fat legs baby," and another said, "Big ass." I felt so embarrassed, humiliated, but most of all, angry... Who do they think they are and how dare they say that to me, a total stranger? I see the same things happen in nightclubs —not just to me but to other girls with perfectly normal figures.

Allie, 18

I wish I could weigh more and have tried without success. I have a very small bust which I really wish I could change. During high school this worried me the most. I did get teased about this on a few occasions by guys mostly. I still get a little depressed when you see perfectly shaped women on television and in movies and when you hear a guy say something like the first thing that they look at when they meet a girl is her breasts or that they would only go out with a girl with big breasts.

Anonymous, 21

body police. Surround yourself as much as you can with activities and people who celebrate who you are and what you can do. Practise the self-esteem and body-image boosters. Remember that one day you will be able to escape your family. If things get desperate, we may have to institute a helicopter rescue service.

Things to say to the body police

Sometimes ignoring them will help, sometimes it encourages further abuse. Try not to fall into the trap of always returning an insult, as you can just get into a slanging match that teaches them nothing and drives you crazy. Sometimes, however, it might be the only way to drive home your point. Enlist your friends so you can help each other go on the offensive.

Ask yourself not "What can I do to make myself more acceptable?" but "What is the matter with that person that they need to judge me by their own insecurities and standards?" People who are truly happy with themselves never bother to slag off other people. There is always a reason why you are being targeted, and it has nothing to do with you.

Some of these suggested retorts (below) can be used as all-pur-pose responses to any body commentary from someone else, such as, "Are you feeling insecure?," "You wouldn't say that without all your mates around," and "Grow up!"

If you just don't feel safe saying any of these things out loud, make sure you say them to yourself. This can be most satisfying. Laughing or smiling after people insult you can drive them crazy. It's a great way to show you don't take their uninformed judgement seriously.

THEY say:

"You're getting a bit fat" (or disapprovingly, "You're put-ting on weight").

YOU say:

"No, I'm not, I'm just growing."

"No I'm not. What did you say that for?"

"Who asked you?"

"Why are you trying to upset me?"

"What is it you are feeling insecure about?"

"I am not fat, I'm me-shaped."

"I'm growing. Any objections?"

"Anything else? Perhaps you could write it down for me so I don't forget?"

"How kind of you to say so."

"I have no intention of going on a stupid, impossible diet just so you feel that your outdated prejudices are validated by pressuring me into action which would be counterproductive and unhealthy, thereby reinforcing the self-loathing recommended by you and your own fears. So, hey, get a life, dickbrain."

"And you're a real heartthrob."

"A bit fat for you, or a bit fat for me?"

"Why don't you grab your bottom lip and pull it over your head?"

"You have no right to comment on my body."

"Yes, thank you, I have put on weight, and I feel great."

"Thank you."

"I'm not worried about it, so relax."

"I'm sorry, but I don't care what you think."

"Nobody was ever thrown out of bed for being cuddly."

"When I need your opinion to make me feel crappy, I'll let you know."

"You're right. I guess I should become anorexic immediately. Would that be all right?"

"Are you trying to give me an eating disorder?"

"You can get a book from the library to explain what shape women are."

"What makes you so interested in my shape?"

"I'm not getting fat, I'm growing. It's this inevitable thing that happens when you're a teenager, like people hassling you."

"You are quite right. I do not have the body of a 12-year-old boy. Do you have one you're not using?"

"What is this? Body insult hour?"

who asked You?

THEY say:

"Why don't you try the new diet/my new diet/a diet?"

YOU say:

"This is my natural shape. If it offends you, please don't look at it."

"I don't need a diet. I eat healthy food."

"Diets don't work."

"I enjoy my food."

"Because I'm not stupid. I know diets don't work."

"Why don't you mind your own body?"

"This is really boring. Can't we talk about something else?"

"I don't want to get obsessed with food."

"I'm happy the way I am."

"Why do you want to run my life?"

"Why do you want to ruin my life?"

"Allow me to get away from you."

"What makes you so interested in my body?"

"Strangely enough, I don't have time to go to the gym for
    five hours a day. Will I be arrested?"

"What's your problem?"

"Do I look that stupid?"

YAWN!

THEY say:

**"You're a real skinny stick, aren't you? Have you got
    anorexia?"**

YOU say:

"Is it my turn to criticise your body now? No."

"Who asked you?"

"Is there anything else you'd like to comment on? Should I
    take notes?"

"Thanks for that, Einstein."

"Cat got your brain?"

"I am naturally thin. You know, like you're naturally rude."

"You mean I'm *thin*? Oh my God, I'd never noticed!"

"Small, but perfectly formed."

"Good things come in small packages."

"I am not a stick. I am a woman, with feelings."

THEY say:

"You've got no tits."

YOU say:

"Well, they're bigger than your brain."

"Your fly is undone."

"What's up your nose?"

"How long have you been looking at me?"

"That's not what you said last night in bed."

"Feeling insecure?"

"Am I supposed to care what you think?"

"What makes you interested in my breasts?"

"Thank you for your intellectual contribution."

"Dang, I knew I forgot something when I got dressed this
     morning."

"Get a life."

"You sound like a three-year-old."

THEY say:
   "Hey, check out the big hooters on that one" or
     "Show us your tits."

YOU say:
"Show us your brain."

Anything in a language they don't understand.

"Don't you know what they look like?"

"Grow up."

"You can always tell a bottle-fed baby."

"There's a big booger coming out of your nose."

"Never mind, when you grow up, a girl might show you what
     breasts look like."

"Why are you so interested in my breasts?"

*An assertiveness-training teacher tells me that this is a good method of
     preserving dignity and (we hope) making people realise how stupid
     they are being. Follow these four simple steps: Stand or sit up
     straight. Pause for at least three seconds. Make firm eye contact. Use
     a well-modulated voice to ask your question or make your state-
     ment. For example:*

"You're getting fat." (Pause.) "Am I?"

Or
"Aren't you too thin?" (Pause.) "No."

The Body Police Quiz

1. Someone criticises your appearance. You immediately think:

(a) I wonder what they're insecure about?

(B) Right, that's it, I'm going to have my head removed.

(c) You might have left the iron on.

2. A guy in the street yells out: "Hey, big ass!" You say:

(a) Excuse me, I think you might have dropped your IQ.

(b) Is that an eel coming out of your nose?

(c) What an attractive human being. That's the sort of man I really admire and like to be around. How about a date?

3. Your mother tells you you should lose some weight. You reply:

(a) Shall I amputate a leg?

(b) I'll start starving myself for your sake, shall I?

(c) Mum, I think you should read this stuff about why diets don't work.

you look weird

4. Your family has been getting at you to lose weight. You call a family meeting and say:

(a) We've got three choices. You stop hassling me, I get bulimia, or you pay for me to go and live in the Bahamas. What'll it be?

(b) This is the shape I am. Your constant nagging does not take account of the fact that diets do not work, I am supposed to look like this, and you're driving me into becoming a neurotic, obsessed, miserable person. I just want to check with you if that's the whole point of this, in which case I am putting in an application to join another family. The Simpsons appeal.

(c) Either you accept me the way I am or I'm going to make extra pocket money by conducting guided tours of the family room of a dysfunctional family.

5. An uncle tells you you have started getting fat. You:

(a) Ask what it has to do with him.

(b) Tell him you could lend him a book on biology which would explain.

(c) Laugh at him.

6. A friend asks you to go on a diet with her. You reply:

(a) Only if it has Mars Bars, broccoli, pumpkin, and custard in it.

(b) Thanks, but I can get bored at the same rate by watching paint dry.

(c) I'll race you to 30 pounds and the first one there's dead, nyah nyah nyah. Oh.

7. A girlfriend says, "I'm so fat. I can't have lunch." You react by:

(a) Explaining that if she doesn't have lunch she'll be inhaling chocolate by 3 P.M.

(b) Saying "You are not fat. That's flesh. It's for holding your bones in."

(c) Who told you that? Come, we shall firebomb them.

8. You have always remembered the guy at school who said your nose is too big. You take comfort from the fact that:

(a) The guy is now living alone in a trailer in Lubbock, Texas, with a part-time job as a sewage sorter.

(b) He was only saying it to impress his mates, who collectively are as attractive to you as a four-hour documentary on the mating frenzy of cane toads.

(c) You have now moved on to a world unpopulated by smelly, 14-year-old boys who have the social skills of a ferret on drugs. He has asked you out three times.

chapter *seven*

In short

There are millions of gorgeous body shapes.
Yours is one of them.
Dieting doesn't work.
Your thighs are pretty cute.
Exercise should be fun not duty.
Expensive cosmetics may not be better than cheapies.
Advertising lies.
Plastic surgery sucks.
Modelling can be miserable.
You can recover from an eating disorder.
You can read magazines and watch television critically.
You can fight the body police.
You are not your buttocks.

the ♥ end
(time for afternoon tea)

Contacts

Women's Information and Referral Centres

For general advice on services available to women and referral to appropriate organisations.

National Organization for Women (NOW)
1000 16th Street NW
Suite 700
Washington, D.C. 20036
Phone: (202)331-0066

Clearinghouse on Women's Issues
P.O. Box 70603
Friendship Heights, MD 20813
Phone: (202)362-3789 or (301)871-6106

National Council of Negro Women
1667 K Street NW
Washington, D.C. 20006
Phone: (202)659-0006

The National Council for Research on Women
530 Broadway
10th floor
New York, NY 10012
Phone: (212)274-0730

Women's Health Care Centres

For help in locating services and finding support groups and information about medical conditions. Call the relevant numbers to find local contacts in your district or town.

Women's Health Initiative
National Institutes of Health
Office of Disease Prevention
Building No. 1, Room 260
9000 Rockville Pike
Bethesda, MD 20289
Phone: (800)549-6636
(You can participate in the WHI's studies of women's health by calling or writing.)

National Women's Health Network
135 G Street, NW
Washington, D.C. 20005
Phone: (202)347-1140

Boston Women's Health Book Collective
240A Elm Street
Somerville, MA 02144
Phone: (617)625-0271

Federation of Feminist Health Centers
633 E. 11th Street
Eugene, OR 97401
Phone: (503)344-0966

National Women's Health Resource Center
2440 M Street, NW
Suite 325
Washington, D.C. 20037
Phone: (202)293-6045

Women's Health Education Project
2271 Second Avenue
New York, NY 10035
Phone: (212)987-0066

Women's Health Resource Center
Brigham and Women's Hospital
850 Boylston Street and Route 9
Chestnut Hill, MA 02167
Phone: (800)522-8765

Women's Self-Help Center
2838 Olive Street
St Louis, MO 63103
Phone: (314)531-2003

Natural Therapies

Traditional herbal medicine is being revived and expanded. People seek these alternative therapies when "modern" medicine has failed, or they combine "modern" medicine and natural remedies.

The most common ailments treated by natural therapists include reproductive and menstrual problems, fatigue, the immune system and recurring conditions (such as thrush), and many chronic respiratory conditions and digestive disorders.

All natural therapists, including practitioners of traditional Chinese medicine, homoeopaths, and herbalists, work with the body as a whole and have an emphasis on prevention.

Beware of the rare sort of hippy-dippy, so-called natural therapists who might claim that a decent dose of pollen juice will make an amputated leg grow back. You can check that your practitioner is accredited with a reputable organisation:

The American Holistic Medical Association
2727 Fairview Avenue East
Seattle, WA 98102
Phone: (206)322-6842

The International Association of Holistic Health Practitioners
3419 Thom Boulevard
Las Vegas, NV 89106
Phone: (712)873-4542

Further reading

Patsy Westcott and Leyardia Black, *Alternative Health Care for Women* (Rochester, Vermont: Thorsons Publishing Group, 1987)

Sporting Bodies

For advice on opportunities in sport access and facilities.

American Alliance for Health, Physical Education, Recreation and Dance
1900 Association Drive
Reston, VA 22091
Phone: (703)476-3450

Women's Sports Foundation
Eisenhower Park
East Meadow, NY 11554
Phone: (800)227-3988

National Collegiate Athletic Association
Education Services Group
6201 College Boulevard
Overland Park, KS 66211
Phone: (913)339-1906

Also contact the Department of Parks and Recreation in your city or state.

Civil Rights and Equal Opportunity Organisations

A good place to start if you have queries regarding discrimination or sexual harassment.

Commission on Civil Rights
1121 Vermont Avenue, NW
Washington, D.C. 20425
Phone: (202)523-5571

Equal Employment Opportunity Commission
7 World Trade Center
18th floor
New York, NY 10047
Phone: (800)669-4000 or (800)669-3302 (deaf access)
(The commission also has offices in most states.)

ACLU Women's Rights Project
American Civil Liberties Union
132 W. 43rd Street
New York, NY 10036
Phone: (212)944-9800

NOW Legal Defense and Education Fund
99 Hudson Street
12th floor
New York, NY 10013
Phone: (212)925-6635

Women's Legal Defense Fund
1875 Connecticut Avenue, NW
Suite 710
Washington, D.C. 20009
Phone: (202)986-2600

Office of Civil Rights
U.S. Department of Education
330 C Street, SW
Washington, D.C. 20202
Phone: (202)708-5366

The Office of Civil Rights deals with sex discrimination against students and employees of federally funded bodies such as educational institutions. You can ask for information or file a complaint at one of these regional offices:

Region 1: Connecticut, Maine, Massachusetts, New Hampshire, Rhode Island, Vermont

JW McCormack Post Office and Courthouse Building
Room 222, 01-0061
Boston, MA 02109
Phone: (617)223-9662

Region 2: New Jersey, New York, Puerto Rico, Virgin Islands
26 Federal Plaza
33rd floor
Room 33-130, 02-1010
New York, NY 10278
Phone: (212)264-5180

Region 3: Delaware, District of Columbia, Maryland, Pennsylvania,
Virginia, West Virginia
3535 Market Street
Room 6300, 03-2010
Philadelphia, PA 19104
Phone: (215)596-6772

Region 4: Alabama, Florida, Georgia, Mississippi, North Carolina,
South Carolina, Tennessee
P.O. Box 2048, 04-3010
Atlanta, GA 30301
Phone: (404)331-2954

Region 5: Illinois, Indiana, Michigan, Minnesota, Ohio, Wisconsin
401 South State Street
Room 700C, 05-4010
Chicago, IL 60605
Phone: (312)886-3456

Region 6: Arkansas, Louisiana, Oklahoma, Texas
1200 Main Tower Building
Suite 2260, 06-5010
Dallas, TX 75202
Phone: (214)767-3959

Region 7: Iowa, Kansas, Kentucky, Missouri, Nebraska
10220 North Executive Hills Boulevard
8th floor, 07-6010
Kansas City, MO 64153
Phone: (816)891-8026

Region 8: Arizona, Colorado, Montana, New Mexico, North Dakota, South Dakota, Utah, Wyoming
Federal Office Building
1961 Stout Street
Room 342, 08-7010
Denver, CO 80294
Phone: (303)844-5695

Region 9: California
Old Federal Building
50 United Nations Plaza
Room 239, 09-8010
San Francisco, CA 94102
Phone: (415)556-7000

Region 10: Alaska, American Samoa, Guam, Hawaii, Idaho, Nevada, Oregon, Washington
915 Second Avenue
Room 3310, 10-9010
Seattle, WA 98174
Phone: (206)442-6811

Cancer Organisations

For information about breast self-examination, lumps and cancer and how to find an appropriate support group.

American Cancer Society
1599 Clifton Road, NE
Atlanta, GA 30329
Phone: (404)320-3333

National Cancer Institute
Department of Health and Human Services
Building 31, Room 10-A24
9000 Rockville Pike
Bethesda, MD 20892
Phone: (301)496-4000

Susan G. Komen Breast Cancer Foundation
Occidental Tower
5005 LBJ Freeway
Suite 370, LB 74
Dallas, TX 75244
Phone: (800)462-9273

Strang-Cornell Breast Center
428 E. 72nd Street
New York, NY 10021
Phone: (212)639-5200

Women's Comprehensive Cancer Screening Program
Duke University Medical Center
P.O. Box 3814
Durham, NC 27710
Phone: (919)684-3785

Women's Cancer Resource Center
3023 Shattuck Avenue
Berkeley, CA 94705
Phone: (415)548-9272

Breast Cancer Network
Mid-America Cancer Center
1235 East Cherokee
Springfield, MO 65804
Phone: (800)432-2273

Y-Me National Organization for Breast Cancer Information and
Support
18220 Harwood Avenue
Homewood, IL 60430
Phone: (708)799-8338 or (708)799-8228
(24-hour hotline)

Environmental Groups

These organisations work against pesticides and toxic chemicals in
our environment.

Mothers and Others for a Livable Planet
40 W. 20th Street
New York, NY 10011
Phone: (212)727-4474

Northwest Coalition for Alternatives to Pesticides
P.O. Box 1393
Eugene, OR 97440
Phone: (503)344-5044

Women's Environment and Development Organization
845 Third Avenue
15th floor
New York, NY 10022
Phone: (212)759-7982

Safe Sex & Planned Parenthood Federation Headquarters

You still need condoms if you're in love: condoms are not just for casual relationships or one-night stands.

If you are having sex—even once—you can get pregnant. Condoms are the only contraception which will prevent pregnancy and also guard against sexually transmitted diseases.

Some places you can hide condoms so they won't fall out include where you hide your tampons; in a cassette tape cover or CD cover; in a small purse with a zip or fold over the flap.

Here are some things you can say to get a guy to wear a condom:

I don't want to get pregnant.

I can't take the Pill: it makes me nauseous.

Please do it for me.

You look lovely in a hat.

If you don't wear a condom I won't do it with you.

Sexually transmitted diseases

One or both of you might be carrying diseases WITHOUT knowing it, as the symptoms are not always obvious, and sometimes mostly happen inside you. Some of them are incurable, some may develop to infertility or cancer, but almost ALL of them are easily cured if treated early.

A guy can be infected with something and never know he has it. In this way, diseases can be passed on silently, without anyone knowing. Some sexually transmitted diseases have "silent" symptoms-for example, no visible sores or warts, or a symptom that could be mistaken for flu or period pains. And if not treated, some diseases will make you infertile.

Common sexually transmitted diseases include chlamydia, the wart virus, herpes, HIV (the AIDS virus), syphilis, gonorrhoea, and some forms of hepatitis.

Further reading

Kaz Cooke, *The Modern Girl's Guide to Safe Sex* (Melbourne: McPhee Gribble, 1993)-Yes, I am flogging my own book

Sherman J. Silber, *How Not to Get Pregnant* (New York: Warner Books, 1990)

For advice on contraception, Pap smear tests, pregnancy, and abortion contact Planned Parenthood and get details from your local clinic:

Planned Parenthood Federation of America, Inc.
810 Seventh Avenue
New York, NY 10019
Phone: (212)603-4600 or (800)248-7797

National Family Planning and Reproductive Health Association
122 C Street, NW
Suite 380
Washington, D.C. 20001
Phone: (202)628-3533

National Organization of Adolescent Pregnancy and Parenting
4421A East-West Highway
Bethesda, MD 20814
Phone: (301)913-0378

Preventing Adolescent Pregnancy
Girls, Inc.
30 E. 33rd Street
New York, NY 10016
Phone: (212)689-3700

Alcohol and Drug Foundations

Contact details are given for sources of information and counselling and referral centres.

National Council on Alcoholism and Drug Dependence
12 W. 21st Street
8th floor
New York, NY 10010
Phone: (800)423-4673 or (212)206-6770

Women's Alcohol and Drug Education Project
370 Lexington Avenue
Suite 603
New York, NY 10017
Phone: (212)532-8330

Woman to Woman
Association of Junior Leagues
660 First Avenue
New York, NY 10016
Phone: (212)683-1515

Women for Sobriety
P.O. Box 618
Quakerstown, PA 18951
Phone: (800)333-1606 or (215)536-8026

Drug Abuse Information Line
Phone: (800)522-5353

Emergency Counselling

You can ring and discuss your problem, at any time of the day or night. The National Directory of Hotlines and Crisis Centers can help you find the right place to handle your type of problem; their phone number is (212)727-4025. Here are the phone numbers of some of the many centres.

Covenant House Nineline: (800)999-9999

National Food Addiction Hotline: (800)872-0088

Cancer Information Service: (800)4CA-NCER

Teens Tap (Teaching AIDS Prevention); you can speak to other people

your age: (800)234-TEEN

CHOICE Hotline (health problems): (215)985-3300

National AIDS Hotline: (800)342-2437 (English); (800)344-7432 (Spanish); (800)243-7889 (deaf access)

National STD Hotline (sexually transmitted diseases): (800) 227-8922

Abortion Hotline: (800)772-9100

National Hate Crime Reporting Hotline: (800)347-4283

Washington, D.C. Rape Crisis Center Hotline: (202)333-7273

National Family Violence Helpline: (800)222-2000

Stepfamily Association of America: (800)735-0329

American Self-Help Clearinghouse (referrals to any self-help group): (201)625-7101

Notes

Chapter 1 Shapes and Sizes

Amounts of body fat by gender before and after puberty (post-adolescent girls have 20 to 30 percent more fat than boys) from *Body Traps: How to Overcome Your Body Obsessions and Liberate the Real You*, by Dr. Judith Rodin (New York: William Morrow, 1992); Fat on girls and muscle on boys in adolescent years from "Weight as Chronic Stressors in Women (WACS)," by Ilana Attie and J. Brooks Gunn, in a book called *Gender and Stress,* edited by Barnett, Biener, and Baruch (London: The Free Press, 1992); Girls who mature early share shorter characteristics research by Faust 1977 quoted in Barnett, Biener, and Baruch, op. cit.; Ballet dancers delaying menstruation by average of three years by M. P. Warren, and below 20 percent body fat as average point that periods stop, quoted by Dr. Ronald Laura and Dr. Christina Lee in *Nature and Health* magazine, Vol. 12, No. 3, August 1991; Age of menstruation onset from *Everygirl* by Derek Llewellyn Jones and Suzanne Abraham (Melbourne: Oxford University Press,1989);"Is Body Fat Distribution Changed by Dieting?" by John Garrow, Department of Human Nutrition, St. Bartholomew's Hospital, London, reported in *Acta Med. Scandinavian Suppl.* 723, pp. 199-203; Hip, thigh, buttock fat harder to shift from "Can Body Fat Patterning Be Changed" *Acta Med. Scandinavian Suppl* 1988, 723; Dr. Sandra Cabot, author of *The Body Shaping Diet,* quoted in *Who Weekly*, 25 October 1993; U.K. *Slimmer* magazine article "You Can Change Your Shape," Oct.-Nov. 1992; Sizes from U.S. Department of Commerce; 1942 measurements, Frances Dysart quotation, American Standards and Testing Materials survey from "Go Figure: Same Shopper Wears 6,8,10,12," by Teri Agins, article in *Wall Street Journal*, 11 November 1994; Interview with Professor Johnson in December 1994; *Being Fat Is Not a Sin*, by Shelley Bovey (London: Pandora, 1989); Historical theory of thin becoming fashionable in the 1920s from Bennett and Gurin 1982 quoted in Barnett, Biener, and Baruch, op. cit.; *Backlash: The Undeclared War Against Women,* by Susan Faludi (New York: Crown, 1991), and *The Beauty Myth,* by Naomi Wolf (New York: William Morrow, 1991); Prejudice against the obese research by Wooley and Wooley 1979 quoted in "Weight as Chronic Stressors in Women (WACS)," Barnett, Biener, and Baruch, reported in the *Utne Reade* magazine, May-June 1992; *Utne Reader* magazine special issue "War on the Body," May-June 1992; Australian Bureau of Statistics figures from *Women in Australia*, ABS Catalogue No 4113.0, method on application to the ABS (their source is the National Health Survey 1989-90; definitions of average, overweight, underweight, and obese applied in the ABS study came from the National Health and Medical Research Council and the National Heart Foundation; Overweight defined as above the 85th percentile from *New England Journal of Medicine,*Vol. 327, No. 19, p. 1379; Waist-Hip ratio information from paper "Self-

Reported Weight and Height in Adolescents and Their Parents," a study by Tienboon, Walqvist, and Rutishauer in the *Journal of Adolescent Health*, 1992, No. 13; Body fat in relation to menstruation and shop mannequin from "Could Mannequins Menstruate," a study by Rinalta and Mustajoki, Dept. of Medicine, University of Central Hospital, Scandinavia.

Chapter 2 Weight for Me

Food
"Shapescope" astrology column in U.K. *Slimmer* magazine, Oct.-Nov. 1992; *Cleo* survey about women and guilt about eating, May 1992, republished July 1993; *Who Weekly*, "Diet Winners and Sinners of the Year," 10 January 1994; Cindy Crawford quotes on dessert in Australian *Cosmopolitan*, March 1993; Interview with Jennifer Saunders in *Mode* magazine, Aug.-Sept. 1993; Mirabella magazine health survey, February 1993; *Understanding Anorexia and Obesity*, by Peter Dally and Joan Gomez (London: Faber and Faber, 1990); Margaret O'Sullivan's book *The Heavenly Body Diet* (Sydney: Pan Macmillan, 1993) reported in the *Sunday Telegraph*, 15 August 1993.
  Nutrition Top-selling supermarket products from Information Resources Inc, a Chicago-based market-research company; Americans eat almost 22 billion fast-food meals from Technomics Inc, another Chicago market-research company; The Victorian Health Promotion Foundation's ideas for healthier eating from Penelope Goward's guide to eating from *Body Image and Eating Awareness Professional Training Manual* for developing groups for adult women, Victorian Health Promotion Foundation, March 1993; South Australia's recommendations from Marion Duff, nutritionist and dietician at Royal Prince Alfred Hospital, Sydney, 1993; Magazine suggesting leaving one of three options on your plate, *Cleo*, March 1993 in "Those Last Three Kilos"; Osteoporosis link to excess animal protein consumption in *Diet for a New America* (see reading list for this section) with information from many sources, including studies of Americans, Bantus, and Eskimos, and papers including "Protein-Induced Hypercalcuria: A Longer-Term Study," by I. Allen, in the *American Journal of Clinical Nutrition*, 1979; "The Effects of Vegetable and Animal Protein Diets on Calcium, Urate and Oxalate Excretion," by J. Brockis, *British Journal of Urology*, 1982, and *Osteoporosis*, by V. Barzel (New York: Grune & Stratton,1970); Physical activity linked to low osteoporosis from *Choice* magazine April 1992.

Dieting
U.S. diet figures from "28 Questions About Fat" in *Life* magazine, February 1995; All quotes from Penelope Goward, nurse, counsellor, and body-image and eating consultant, taken from the *Age*, 4 April 1990; Obesity report showing 95 percent recidivist rate by dieters published by the Royal College of Physicians of London in their own journal, Vol. 17, No. 1, January 1983, quoted in *Being Fat Is Not a Sin* by Shelley Bovey (London: Pandora,1989); Texas study and quotes from Karen Carrier from the *Sunday Age*, 5 January 1992; Dr. Jane Ogden quoted in *Health and Fitness* magazine, October 1992; *Don't Diet*, by Dr. Dale Atrens (New York: Bantam,1988); Study of 55 English students including 13 dieters reported in *Sydney Morning Herald*, 17 December 1992; Dieting fourth-graders from *Life* magazine, February 1995; Quotes on children and adolescents dieting from Ms. Jenny O'Dea and Dr. Mark Walqvist from the *Sydney Morning Herald*, 4 June 1993; U.S. diet figures from *Life* magazine, February 1995; Interviews with dietician Jo Rogers in *Who Weekly* magazine, 22 March 1993; National Heart Foundation condemns fad "heart" diets, *Aus-*

tralian Doctor magazine, 16 July 1993; *The Weight Loss Guide* by the National Heart Foundation is given free to inquirers and is available at health centres (ISBN 1-875545-11-5); *Choice* magazine survey of weight-loss programs, June 1993; *Sunday Age* reporter misled by weight-loss centres in the *Sunday Age,* 22 August 1993; Consumer Advocacy and Financial Counselling Association investigation of weight-loss centres reported in the *Sunday Age,* 22 December 1992; U.S. diet program spending from *Life* magazine, February 1995; A reader's story in *Dolly* magazine about addiction to diet pills, February 1993; Worry from doctors on overprescription of diet pills from Professor Paul Zimmet of the Australian Society for the Study of Obesity in the *Sunday Age,* 25 July 1993; *Dolly* criticises liquid diets, February 1993; U.S. National Institutes of Health report quoted by Greer Kessel in *Allure* magazine, 1993; U.K. *Slimmer* magazine, problem pages, Oct.-Nov. 1992; Dr. Jane Ogden quoted in *Health and Fitness* magazine, October 1992; American women now eating what they like and U.S. diet statistics from the *Bulletin* magazine, 25 August 1992.

Obesity
Definition of obese as over 30 on body mass index from the National Health Survey, 1990, Australian Bureau of Statistics; 33.4 per cent of adults overweight from Robert J Kuczmarski et al., "Increasing Prevalence of Overweight among U.S. Adults," *Journal of the American Medical Association*, 20 July 1994, Vol. 272, no 3; Anne Marie Droulers, a psychologist from Royal Prince Alfred Hospital, from *Cleo* magazine, 1993; Comments from Penelope Goward and obesity conference from the *Age,* 15 September 1993; Research interview with Susan Thompson, dietician from the Royal Alexandria Hospital for Children, Camperdown, 1994; Obese U.S. school students from *Life*, February 1995; Dr. Court's comments and study on overweight high school students reported in the *Age,* 8 June 1993; "Psychosocial Factors in Obesity," a paper by Dr. Perlli Mustajoki, University of Helsinki, Finland, published in *Annals of Clinical Research* , Vol.19, 1987, pp. 143-46; The Body Image and Eating Behaviour Project, Victoria Health Promotion Foundation; Details of obesity from *The New A to Z of Women's Health: A Concise Encyclopaedia,* by Christine Animer (Alameda, CA: Hunter House Inc, 1989); Obese may remain obese without overeating research by Stunkard, Sorenson, and others, 1986, quoted in the chapter "Weight as Chronic Stressors in Women(WACS)," Barnett, Biener, and Baruch, op. cit.;

Eating Disorders
Interview with Dr. Peter Clark from the Royal Prince Alfred Hospital Eating Disorders Clinic, 1993; U.S. eating disorder figures from National Association of Anorexia Nervosa and Associated Disorders brochure, "Compelling Reasons to Intensify and Expand Eating Disorders Prevention and Education Programs"; La Trobe University study results from article in the *Sunday Age,* 7 January 1993; Definitions and causes of anorexia and bulimia from the Royal Prince Alfred Hospital Eating Disorders Clinic information kit; Some description of symptoms of anorexia and bulimia from Dr. Janice Russell, University of Sydney lecturer and eating-disorders authority, Sydney, in *Australian Doctor,* 30 August 1991; Experiences of anorexics Tracey Gold and Karen Carpenter from *Cleo,* August 1992; Julie Dickinson of Perth Eating-Disorders Clinic warns that private schoolgirls are highly represented in anorexia programs, *Sydney Morning Herald,* 8 October 1993; Dr. Suzanne Abraham's article "Anorexia, Bulimia Update," *Sydney Morning Herald,* 7 July 1990; Gym school established at Fairfield West Primary School, *Sydney Morning Herald,* 9 July 1993; Jeff Bond, head of sports psychology at the Australian Institute of Sport, quoted on anorexia and elite sport in the *Sydney Morning Herald,* 15 December 1992; Jeff Bond interviewed on gymnasts' school and helping athletes under training, 5 January 1994; Information on ballet dancers from quotes by Professor Beumont, Psychiatry Dept., Sydney University, in a *Sydney Morning Herald* article, 5 June 1993; *Age* letters from

Melborne psychiatrist Dr Jerome Gelb, 20 July 1993, and from McArthur and MacLeod, 2 April 1993; *Vogue* editor's comments in article from *The Independent*, republished in the *Age*, 1993; No women's magazines in eating-disorder clinics article in the *Melbourne Weekly*, May 1993; Families and friends suggestions from Royal Prince Henry Hospital eating-disorders clinic.

Exercise
Women's exercise statistics from "Girls Don't Want to Have Gym," by Jennifer Steinhauer, *New York Times* article, 4 January 1995; U.S. phys ed classes from *Life* magazine, February 1995; The Australian School Fitness Test 1986 results, Pyke, quoted in the *Active Girls Can Do Anything Kit* schools education campaign kit citing fitness statistics provided by the Federal Department of Sport, Education and Training (the kit is produced by the Australian Sports Commission and the National Heart Foundation); Stoddart's 1993 report on women, sport, and the media in the *Australian Sports Directory*, 1993; U.S. girls and sports figures from National Federation of State High School Associations; Anorexia linked to overexercise article quoting Professor Peter Beumont, *Sydney Morning Herald,* 11 September 1993; Ballet dancers prone to anorexia and bulimia says Professor Peter Beumont and Virginia Gallagher quotes from *Sydney Morning Herald*, 5 June 1993; Kirkland and Morris quotes in U.S. *Self* magazine, April 1992; *Cleo* magazine quoting Dr. Stuart Watson of the Australian College of Sports Physicians on endurance runners, March 1993; *Allure* magazine exercise special, June 1993; Exercise benefits from the *Sydney Morning Herald* article on Australians getting fatter younger, 8 September 1993.

Chapter 3 What Is Normal?

Breasts
Breastman Denis Leary's comments from his book *No Cure for Cancer* (New York: Anchor Books, 1992; it's also available on CD or cassette from A&M Records); Breast lumps, cancer, and examination from New South Wales Cancer Council information and research interview with Germana Morassi, health promotions officer, Breast X-ray Program, Rachel Forster Hospital, Redfern, New South Wales; U.S. breast cancer figures from National Cancer Institute; breast cancer gene from Gayle Feldman, "When Women Know Too Much," *New York Times*, 12 October 1994; High-fibre diet link to low breast cancer risk from CSIRO study of 902 Adelaide women reported in *Sydney Morning Herald*, 9 March 1994; Environmental links to breast cancer from the *Utne Reader* Nov.-Dec. 1993 and *Ms.* magazine special issue on breasts, May-June 1993; Inverted nipples, U.K. *Marie Claire* magazine, June and July 1993; Instructional tape transcript, *Harper's* magazine, May 1993; *Vogue* announced small breasts are back on the cover, April 1993; Wonderbra craze in the *Weekly Telegraph*, No. 108, 4 October 1993; Sports bra sports medicine advice, *Allure* magazine November 1992; Letter from Dr. Edward Ryan to the *Medical Journal of Australia* about pain caused by bra straps; Large breasts special in U.K. *Marie Claire* magazine, February 1993.

Thighs, Stretch Marks, and the Cellulite Scam
Cover-lines series from *Cleo* magazine, September 1993; Apology in November issue; $130 million spent on cellulite in U.S. and quotes from Drs. Basler, Shulman, Bailey and Matarasso all from U.S. *Glamour* magazine, October 1993; "No Cream

Will Restore Elasticity to Your Skin," Dr. Helen Cole, U.S. *Glamour*, February 1993; U.K. *Marie Claire* magazine, cellulite beauty special, 1993; "Body sculpture" article in *Follow Me* magazine, July1990, listing treatments and products; Stretch marks, *Australian Doctor* magazine, 15 January 1993.

Periods
Amount of average flow, *Choice* magazine tampon survey and safety check, April 1992; Blue ink on pad, Whisper TV advertisement screened 1993-4; Article on PMS in *Elle* magazine, February 1993; PMS self-help remedies from Leichardt Women's Community Health Centre literature and *The New Our Bodies Ourselves* by the Boston Women's Health Book Collective (New York: Touchstone Books, 1992); *Choice* magazine PMS treatments survey, October 1991; Overall information provided by Ruth Trickey, naturopath, Western and Chinese herbalist, acupuncturist, and midwife, from the Clifton Hill Natural Health Centre, Melbourne, and *Everywoman's Medical Handbook*, by Dr. Miriam Stoppard (Melbourne: Penguin, 1989).

Skin
Everywoman's Medical Handbook, by Dr. Miriam Stoppard, op.cit.; Acne article, *Sydney Morning Herald*, 1 October 1993; Australian Cancer Council information; U.S. skin cancer figures and precautions from National Cancer Institute, *American Cancer Society Cancer Facts & Figures 1994*, p. 15; Skin cancer special, *Fashion Quarterly*, Summer 1992; Research interview with Dr. Alan Cooper, Australian College of Dermatologists, 1993; Fake tanning article in the *Age* fashion section, p. 2, December 1992; Clipping from *Cosmopolitan* on skin lightening.

Smells
The difference between deodorants and antiperspirants, *Top Sante*magazine, June 1993.

Cosmetic Surgery
Quotes from *Everywoman's Medical Handbook*, by Dr. Miriam Stoppard, op.cit.; The *Sun*'s "Give Yourself a Lift" article, 28 March 1989; Sugeons and clinics, information sheets carrying descriptions of procedures and convalescence given to customers by the Heber Davis clinic, Annandale, Sydney, 1993; Clinics which advertise often inferior, *Sunday Age,* 19 Jan 1992; Quotes from liposuction customers who have displaced fat and had terrible pain, *Fashion Quarterly,* Summer 1993; Liposuction customer Judith Newman's story in *Mode*, Oct.-Nov. 1992; Saline implants information in brochure from Dr. Leo Rozner's practice; Silly Putty comparison by Barbara Erenreich in *Time* magazine, 17 February 1992; 2 million American women have had breast implants in *Backlash: The Undeclared War Against Women*, by Susan Faludi, op. cit.; Dow Corning rat tests in Australian *Vogue*, August 1993; Ron Laura wrote for *Nature and Health*, February 1993; Number of lawsuits filed from "FDA and AMA Clash on Breast Implants," *Washington Post*, 1 December 1994; Statistics on implants from "3 Companies in Landmark Accord on Lawsuits Over Breast Implants," *New York Times*, 24 March 1994; Breast Implant Litigation Fund from "Breast-Implant Ruling Aids Aliens' Claims," *New York Newsday*, 10 August 1994; Specific terms of the Litigation Fund, "What Accord Would Mean for Women with Implants," *New York Times*, 24 March 1994; U.S. collagen costs from the American Society of Plastic and Reconstructive Surgeons; *Cleo* magazine collagen warning, April 1992; Dr. Darryl Hodgkinson on laser surgery in *New Woman* magazine, September 1993; quotes from research interviews with Dr. Leo Rozner, plastic surgeon, 1993, and Dr. Rozner's *Avenue Cosmetic Plastic Surgery Health Update* newsletters to clients from the same year.

Chapter 4 Fashion Victims

Models and Role Models
Vogue feature on top models of 1988 quoted in *Being Fat Is Not a Sin*, by Shelley Bovey (London: Pandora Press,1989); Cindy Crawford's weight-for-height statistics, *Diet and Lifestyle* magazine, Oct.-Nov. 1992; Cindy Crawford quote, *Who Weekly,* 19 March 1993; *Cleo*'s reporter at the New York fashion shows, August 1993; oft-reported unsourced Linda Evangelista quote "We don't get out of bed for less than $10,000 a day"; Elle Macpherson book quote from *Sydney Morning Herald Good Weekend* magazine, 3 October 1993; Lynn Snowden quoted in *Esquire* magazine article on modelling by Philip Weiss, July 1993; Another top agent told *New York* magazine, July 1993; Tanya Arpadi's eating habits, *Dolly* magazine cover-model contest 1993; *Cleo* article on "snotty stringbean"waifs, September 1993; Model characteristics in clipping from *Cosmopolitan* clipping; Emma Balfour and Kate Moss,in *Who Weekly,* 19 July 1993; Richard Harper, a director of Cameron's modelling agency, quoted in *Living Well* magazine, Spring 1993; *Harper's Bazaar* article on waifs, July 1993; Research interview, 1993 and Australian *Vogue* interview, June 1993, with Penelope Tree; *Cleo* horrified by waifs, September 1993; Interview with Eileen Ford in *Sun Herald,* August 1993; Research interview with Dianne Parks, U.K. *Slimming* magazine's Australian editor; *Who Weekly* article with quotes from Beverly Johnson, Carol Alt, and Kim Alexis, 7 December 1992; Carlotta Moye, *Dolly,* research interview 1994; Victoria Collison, *Vogue,* research interview, 1994; Catherine Murphy, *Girlfriend,* research interview,1994.

The Fashion Industry
U.S. fashion sales from Department of Commerce Bureau of Economic Analysis, *Survey of Current Business,* April 1995 issue; $975 billion figure from *The Look* television series screened on ABC, 29 April 1993; Bra sales from Susan Faludi, *Backlash* (New York: Crown, 1991) op. cit.; Fashion trends article in the *Bulletin,* 17 August 1993; *Allure* magazine article on the bustier, November 1992; Lee jeans ad in *US* magazine, August 1993.

The Style Police
Cynthia Heimel quote from *Get Your Tongue out of My Mouth, I'm Kissing You Goodbye* (New York: Ballantine,1993); *The Mode Brides Essential Wedding Organiser* (Australian Consolidated Press, no date); The *Sunday Age* article "Dress to Depress: The 50 All-Time Fashion Disasters," 15 August 1993; *Who Weekly* Best and Worst Dressed Issue 1993; Bruce Weber, *The Look* television series broadcast on ABC, 29 April 1993; U.S. *Vogue* ad revenue from *Advertising Age,* 20 June 1994; Handbag story from *D. V.,* Diana Vreeland's biography (New York: Weidenfeld & Nicholson).

Chapter 5 Hyper Hype

Lotions and potions
Cosmetics sales from Department of Commerce Bureau of Economic Statistics, sections: toilet articles and preparation, clothing and shoes, in *Survey of Current Business,* April 1995 issue; Moisturiser surveys in *Choice* magazine, 1986 and December 1991; Report on "anti-ageing cosmetics" ads in *Choice* reported in the *Age,* 15 May 1990; *New Idea* article on new "anti-ageing" breakthroughs, 20 February 1993, and interview with the writer, October 1993; 70 percent of women cleanse face with soap

from *New Woman* magazine, September 1993; Quotes on toning and on beauty page shenanigans from dermatologist Dr. Peter Berger from his book *Skin Secrets* (Sydney: Allen & Unwin, 1991); Clipping from *Ms.* magazine on Princess Marcella Borghese face cream; Cosmetics advertising regulation from Federal Trade Commission in an interview with Leslie Fair, an attorney in the Advertising Practices division; Science-speak advertisements from Australian, U.S., and English women's magazines in 1992 and 1993; Dr. Tony White's analysis of liposome diagram in the *Age*, 15 November 1993; Environmental hazards from the *Washington Post* report of seminar on women's health and the environment reprinted in the *Age*, 30 July 1993; Urban Detox cream endorsed by U.S. *Elle* magazine, June 1993; *New Idea* on ceramides, 20 February 1993; Comprehensive article on ageing and the efficacy of moisturisers and ingredients with quotes from Professor Cleary and Dr. Cooper by Deborah Bogle in the *Australian*, 11 April 1992; Australasian College of Dermatologists and Australian Consumer's Association on Retin-A in *New Idea*, 20 February 1993; Research interview with a spokesman for the federal health department's Adverse Drug Reactions Committee who wishes to remain anonymous, December 1995; *The Lancet*, 14 March 1992, on birth defects; The letter from Janssen Cilag to doctors and pharmacists dated 5 July 1993; FDA on Retin-A in *Glamour*, May 1991; Cosmetics labelling from Federal Drug Administration; "French" ads similarly collected from various magazines translated by Janet Hall; Seaweed claims U.S. *Madamoiselle* magazine, October 1993; Safety in cosmetics information from "Making Cosmetics Companies Accountable" article in the *Age*, 10 October 1990; Professor Duggin's worries about cosmetic toxicology reported in the *Sun Herald*, 1 August 1993; Urocanic acid recall articles in the *Age*, 20 and 22 December 1990; Natural cosmetics ingredients from *Being Beautiful*, by Zia Wesley (Hosford, Australia: Whatever Publishing Inc., 1983); General information and checking supplied by a representative of the Australasian College of Dermatologists.

Makeup
Choice magazine article on animal testing and alternatives, March 1993; Leaving your makeup bag at home from *Fashion Quarterly*, Summer 1993; Various beauty pages from *Vogue, Allure, Cleo, Mirabella, Dolly, Cosmopolitan*; Flirting hints from *Hair, Body and Beauty*, Winter 1993; Makeup packaging 60 percent of retail cost reported by U.S. *Allure* magazine; New York survey of counter sales pitches, *Glamour* magazine, February 1993; Names of makeup colours from *Mademoiselle*, September 1993; Old mascara causing permanent eye damage risk from *The A to Z of Women's Health: A Concise Encyclopaedia*, by Christine Animer (Alameda, CA: Hunter House Inc., 1989), op. cit.; *The Green Consumer Guide*, by John Elkington (London: Penguin Books, 1989), and Julia Hailes with *Choice* magazine ; Animal testing information from Humane Society of the U.S.

Perfume
History of perfumes in *Let There Be Clothes*, by Lyn Schnurnberger (New York: Workman Publishing,1991); Bathing habits of Elizabeth I and the Duke of Norfolk revealed in *The History of Vanity* by John Woodforde (New York: St Martins Press, 1992); Price of Chanel No. 5 breakdown from *The Look*, screened on ABC television, 29 April 1993; Allergic reactions from *Everywoman's Medical Handbook*, by Dr. Miriam Stoppard, op. cit.; Extract facts from Australian *Vogue*, August 1993; Statistics and launch party details from *Sydney Morning Herald Good Weekend* magazine, 2 October 1993.

Hair
General information from research interview with Mr. David Salinger, spokesperson for the Australian Trichologists Association (hair specialists), 30 November 1993.

Chapter 6 You Are Not Your Buttocks

The Eating Behaviour Manual produced by the Victoria Health Promotion Foundation's Body Image and Eating Behaviour Project, available from the Food and Nutrition Program of the Victorian Health Promotion Foundation; University of New South Wales study on couples and researchers at Flinders University on body image among adults, teenagers and children reported in the *Australian,* 17 November 1990; *Cleo* survey of dieting and women, May 1992; 47 percent of normal-weight women in the U.S. want to be thinner from Lisa Di Mona and Constance Herndon, eds., *The Information Please Women's Sourcebook* (Boston: Houghton Mifflin, 1994); measurements of lingerie models from the *Sunday Age,* 29 November 1992; Twiggy's comments on self-image in *Who Weekly* 1993; Jeff Bond, head of sports psychology at the Australian Institute of Sport, quoted on anorexia and elite sport in *Sydney Morning Herald,* 15 December 1992; 1991 study "Adolescents Problems and Their Relationship to Self-Esteem," by Juliet Harper, from Macquarie University's School of Behavioural Sciences, and Elizabeth Marshall, a counsellor with the New South Wales Department of Education; Comments by Dr. Deborah Saltman and Dr. James Masterton from *The Search for the Real Self: Unmasking the Personality Disorders of Our Age* (New York: Free Press, 1990); Interview with Robin Morgan about *Ms.* magazine and feminism in the Age 10 February 1993; Belly dancer comments from The Sunday *Age,* 29 November 1992; "You can always tell the bottle-fed boys" from comedian Wendy Harmer's stage reply to moronic hecklers saying "Show us your tits"; Assertiveness-training hints from a correspondent to "Keep Yourself Nice," column in the *Age* newspaper, 1990.

Index